# Obstetr
# Gynec

## NOTICE

Medicine is an ever-changing science. As new research and clinical experience broaden our knowledge, changes in treatment and drug therapy are required. The editors and the publisher of this work have made every effort to ensure that the drug dosage schedules herein are accurate and in accord with the standards accepted at the time of publication. Readers are advised, however, to check the product information sheet included in the package of each drug they plan to administer to be certain that changes have not been made in the recommended dose or in the contraindications for administration. This recommendation is of particular importance in regard to new or infrequently used drugs.

# Obstetrics and Gynecology:
## PreTest® Self-Assessment and Review

### Second Edition

## Editor
William H. Swartz, M.D.
Associate Professor of Reproductive Medicine
University of California, San Diego, School of Medicine
La Jolla, California

## Associate Editors
Kiat B. Lim, M.D., F.R.C.S.(c)
Assistant Professor of Reproductive Medicine
University of California, San Diego, School of Medicine
La Jolla, California

John J. Willems, M.D., F.R.C.S.(c)
Assistant Professor of Reproductive Medicine
University of California, San Diego, School of Medicine
La Jolla, California

McGraw-Hill Book Company
Health Professions Division
PreTest Series

*New York St. Louis San Francisco Auckland Bogotá Guatemala Hamburg Johannesburg Lisbon London Madrid Mexico Montreal New Delhi Panama Paris São Paulo Singapore Sydney Tokyo Toronto*

Library of Congress Cataloging in Publication Data
Main entry under title:

Obstetrics and gynecology: PreTest self-assessment and review
  First ed. (1978) edited by A. H. DeCherney.
  Bibliography: p.
  1. Gynecology—Examinations, questions, etc.
  2. Obstetrics—Examinations, questions, etc.
  I. Swartz, William H. II. Willems, John J.
  III. Lim, Kiat B. [DNIM: 1. Obstetrics—
  Examination questions. 2. Gynecology—Examination
  questions. WP 18 014]
  RG111.037  1982   618'.076   80-39952

ISBN 0-07-050975-1

Editor: *Jane Edwards*
Project Editor: *Bruce MacGregor*
Editorial Assistant: *Donna Altieri*
Production: *Rosemary J. Pascale,*
*Judith M. Raccio*
Designer: *Robert Tutsky*
Printer: *Hull Printing Company*
Cover Illustration: *Adapted from photographs of Howard A. Kelly (1858-1943), the first Professor of Obstetrics and Gynecology at The Johns Hopkins Hospital, and Margaret H. Sanger (1893-1966), America's foremost advocate of birth control and founder of the Planned Parenthood Federation.*

Copyright © 1982 1978 by McGraw-Hill, Inc. All rights reserved. Printed in the United States of America. Except as permitted under the Copyright Act of 1976, no part of this publication may be reproduced or distributed in any form or by any means, or stored in a data base or retrieval system, without the prior written permission of the publisher.

3 4 5 6 7 8 9 0  HUHU  8 7 6 5 4 3 2

# Contents

| | |
|---|---|
| Introduction | vii |
| Acknowledgment | ix |

## BIOLOGY AND PHYSIOLOGY OF REPRODUCTION

Anatomy, Genetics, Embryology, and Congenital Anomalies
| | |
|---|---|
| Questions | 3 |
| Answers, Explanations, and References | 9 |

Puberty, Menstruation, Menopause, Sexuality, and Conception
| | |
|---|---|
| Questions | 16 |
| Answers, Explanations, and References | 21 |

Pregnancy, Lactation, and Puerperium
| | |
|---|---|
| Questions | 27 |
| Answers, Explanations, and References | 32 |

## PRIMARY CARE

History, Physical Examination, and Diagnostic Procedures
| | |
|---|---|
| Questions | 40 |
| Answers, Explanations, and References | 46 |

Clinical, Behavioral, Medical, and Legal Problems
| | |
|---|---|
| Questions | 52 |
| Answers, Explanations, and References | 58 |

Contraception, Abortion, and Sterilization
| | |
|---|---|
| Questions | 66 |
| Answers, Explanations, and References | 73 |

## NORMAL PREGNANCY

The Fetus, Placenta, and Newborn
| | |
|---|---|
| Questions | 82 |
| Answers, Explanations, and References | 89 |

Pregnancy, Labor, Delivery, and Puerperium
   Questions     97
   Answers, Explanations, and References     104

## ABNORMALITIES OF PREGNANCY

Spontaneous Abortion, Ectopic Pregnancies, and Trophoblastic Disease
   Questions     112
   Answers, Explanations, and References     118

Medical, Surgical, and Obstetrical Complications of Pregnancy
   Questions     124
   Answers, Explanations, and References     133

Diagnosis and Management of Disorders of Labor, Delivery, and Puerperium
   Questions     145
   Answers, Explanations, and References     151

## CLINICAL GYNECOLOGY

Menstrual and Endocrine Disorders
   Questions     158
   Answers, Explanations, and References     163

Pelvic Relaxation, Infections, Endometriosis, and Infertility
   Questions     169
   Answers, Explanations, and References     179

Benign and Malignant Neoplasms
   Questions     189
   Answers, Explanations, and References     203

**Bibliography**     217

# Introduction

*Obstetrics and Gynecology: PreTest Self-Assessment and Review*, 2nd Ed., has been designed to provide medical students, as well as physicians, with a comprehensive and convenient instrument for self-assessment and review within the field of obstetrics and gynecology. The 500 questions provided have been designed to parallel the format and degree of difficulty of the questions contained in Part II of the National Board of Medical Examiners examinations, the Federation Licensing Examination (FLEX), the Visa Qualifying Examination, and the ECFMG examination.

Each question in the book is accompanied by an answer, a paragraph explanation, and a specific page reference to either a current journal article, a textbook, or both. A four page bibliography, listing all the sources used in the book, follows the last chapter.

Perhaps the most effective way to use this book is to allow yourself one minute to answer each question in a given chapter; as you proceed, indicate your answer beside each question. By following this suggestion, you will be approximating the time limits imposed by the board examinations previously mentioned.

When you finish answering the questions in a chapter, you should then spend as much time as you need verifying your answers and carefully reading the explanations. Although you should pay special attention to the explanations for the questions you answered incorrectly, you should read **every** explanation. The author of this book has designed the explanations to reinforce and supplement the information tested by the questions. If, after reading the explanations for a given chapter, you feel you need still more information about the material covered, you should consult and study the references indicated.

This book meets the criteria for up to 22 credit hours in Category 5(d) for the Physician's Recognition Award of the American Medical Association. It should provide an experience that is instructive as well as evaluative; we also hope that you enjoy it. We would be very happy to receive your comments.

# Acknowledgment

As the editors of the second edition of *Obstetrics and Gynecology: PreTest Self-Assessment and Review*, we would like to acknowledge the contribution of the editors of the first edition, many of whose questions have been retained, albeit modified and updated.

William H. Swartz
Kiat B. Lim
John J. Willems

# BIOLOGY AND PHYSIOLOGY OF REPRODUCTION

# Anatomy, Genetics, Embryology, and Congenital Anomalies

DIRECTIONS: Each question below contains five suggested answers. Choose the one best response to each question.

1. Achondroplasia is best characterized by which of the following statements?

(A) The inheritance pattern is autosomal recessive
(B) Mutation accounts for 80 percent of all cases
(C) Cesarean section is rarely necessary
(D) Affected women rarely live to the reproductive age
(E) None of the above

2. Ambiguous genitalia in 50 percent of all affected infants is caused by

(A) chromosomal nondisjunction
(B) gonadal dysgenesis
(C) adrenal hyperplasia
(D) mosaicism
(E) testicular feminization

3. A 42-year-old woman undergoes a Marshall-Marchetti-Krantz operation for true urinary stress incontinence. The jack-knife position in which the knees are bent and abducted laterally is used during the procedure. Postoperatively, the patient complains of footdrop and loss of sensation on the dorsal aspect of her right foot. The nerve most likely to have been injured during this operation is the

(A) obturator
(B) internal pudendal
(C) common peroneal
(D) ilioinguinal
(E) genitofemoral

4. What is the correct order of the four sections of the fallopian tubes from the ovary to the uterus?
 (A) Ampulla, isthmus, infundibulum, and interstitium
 (B) Interstitium, isthmus, ampulla, and infundibulum
 (C) Interstitium, ampulla, isthmus, and infundibulum
 (D) Infundibulum, isthmus, ampulla, and interstitium
 (E) Infundibulum, ampulla, isthmus, and interstitium

5. The most important indication for surgical repair of a double uterus is
 (A) habitual abortion
 (B) dysmenorrhea
 (C) menometrorrhagia
 (D) dyspareunia
 (E) premature delivery

# Anatomy, Genetics, and Embryology

**DIRECTIONS**: Each question below contains four suggested answers of which **one** or **more** is correct. Choose the answer:

| | | | |
|---|---|---|---|
| A | if | 1, 2, and 3 | are correct |
| B | if | 1 and 3 | are correct |
| C | if | 2 and 4 | are correct |
| D | if | 4 | is correct |
| E | if | 1, 2, 3, and 4 | are correct |

6. A carrier of a balanced 14/21 (D/G) translocation is described by which of the following statements?

(1) Amniocentesis can detect offspring who have translocation Down's syndrome as well as those who are balanced carriers
(2) Karyotype analysis would reveal 45 chromosomes in each cell
(3) Chromosome studies of members of a carrier's family are indicated to detect others at risk for having children with Down's syndrome
(4) The risk for bearing children who have Down's syndrome is the same whether the husband or the wife is the carrier

7. Individuals with the karyotype 45,X are likely to have

(1) a webbed neck, shield chest, high-arched palate, and low-set ears
(2) lymphedema of the extremities at birth
(3) a high incidence of diabetes mellitus
(4) mothers who are over 35 years of age

8. True statements about a pregnant woman who has phenylketonuria include which of the following?

(1) If the father carries the gene, the risk that the child will be affected is 25 percent
(2) If the father carries the gene, amniocentesis and selective abortion can avert the birth of affected children
(3) Individuals with phenylketonuria rarely survive to the reproductive years
(4) Children born to mothers who have phenylketonuria are frequently mentally retarded

9. The karyotypes associated with Turner's syndrome include

(1) 46,XXr
(2) 46,XXp-
(3) 46,Xi(Xq)
(4) 46,X,i(Xp)

## SUMMARY OF DIRECTIONS

| A | B | C | D | E |
|---|---|---|---|---|
| 1, 2, 3 only | 1, 3 only | 2, 4 only | 4 only | All are correct |

10. The advantages of transverse abdominal incisions include

(1) a decreased incidence of incisional hernias
(2) the requirement of only light general anesthesia
(3) a scar that can be cosmetically hidden
(4) easy access to the upper abdomen for bowel surgery

11. A bicornuate uterus (bicornis unicollis) is associated with

(1) failure of complete fusion of the müllerian duct system
(2) an increase in obstetrical complications
(3) an increase in urinary tract anomalies
(4) cervical and vaginal malformations

12. In patients with carcinoma of the vulva, lymphatic drainage characteristically

(1) is to the periaortic nodes
(2) is to the superficial inguinal lymph nodes
(3) bypasses the deep femoral lymph nodes
(4) is from the clitoral region to the deep femoral lymph nodes

13. A group of congenital anomalies known collectively as Potter's syndrome includes renal agenesis (or other renal anomalies) and pulmonary hypoplasia. Other anomalies associated with Potter's syndrome include

(1) hydrocephaly
(2) amnion nodosum
(3) cleft palate
(4) oligohydramnios

14. Diseases that have a positive correlation between maternal infection during pregnancy and congenital anomalies in the fetus include

(1) rubella
(2) mumps
(3) cytomegalovirus
(4) influenza

# Anatomy, Genetics, and Embryology

**DIRECTIONS:** The groups of questions below consist of lettered choices followed by several numbered items. For each numbered item select the **one** lettered choice with which it is **most** closely associated. Each lettered choice may be used once, more than once, or not at all.

## Questions 15-19

For each description that follows, select the blood vessel with which it is most likely to be associated.

(A) Uterine vein
(B) Right ovarian vein
(C) Left ovarian vein
(D) Uterine artery
(E) Ovarian artery

15. Arises from the anterior branch of the hypogastric artery

16. Drains into the internal iliac veins

17. Drains into the inferior vena cava

18. Arises from the abdominal aorta

19. Drains into the left renal vein

## Questions 20-24

For each structure that follows, select its embryological origin.

(A) Genital tubercle
(B) Genital swellings
(C) Urogenital sinus
(D) Urethral folds
(E) Müllerian ducts

20. Labia minora

21. Labia majora

22. Clitoris

23. Vagina

24. Fallopian tubes

## Questions 25-29

Match the following female structures with their male homologues.

(A) Gubernaculum testis
(B) Prostate gland
(C) Scrotum
(D) Vas deferens
(E) Phallus

25. Paraurethral glands

26. Labia majora

27. Round ligament

28. Gartner's duct

29. Clitoris

## Questions 30-34

For each of the following clinical situations, select the most appropriate risk figure.

(A) Equal to that of the U.S. population
(B) 1 percent
(C) 5 percent
(D) 25 percent
(E) None of the above

30. A 21-year-old pregnant woman, whose father had Huntington's chorea and died last year at 47 years of age, wants to know what the chances are that her unborn child will develop the disease. She has been evaluated by a neurologist, who found no evidence of Huntington's chorea

31. A Jewish couple of Ashkenazi ancestry, who are considering having a child, request information about the risk that the child will be born with Tay-Sachs disease

32. A 23-year-old woman has a son with Down's syndrome (47,XY,+21). She wishes to know what the chances are that subsequent children will have the disorder

33. A 27-year-old pregnant woman wants to know if she is at risk for having a child with Down's syndrome. Her 15-year-old sister (47,XX,+21) has the disorder

34. A 26-year-old woman has had one child with spina bifida. During her second pregnancy, prenatal diagnosis detects an open neural tube defect in the fetus. Following termination of that pregnancy, the woman and her husband request information regarding the risk for this disorder in future pregnancies

# Anatomy, Genetics, Embryology, and Congenital Anomalies

# Answers

1. **The answer is B.** *(Burrow, pp 820-821.)* Achondroplasia, a congenital disorder of cartilage formation characterized by dwarfism, is associated with an autosomal dominant pattern of inheritance. However, mutation accounts for 80 percent of all cases of the disorder. Affected women almost always require cesarean section because of the distorted shape of their pelves. Women who have achondroplasia and receive adequate treatment for its associated complications, including the neurological signs of cord compression due to spinal deformity, generally have a normal life expectancy.

2. **The answer is C.** *(Green, ed 3. p 109.)* Although congenital adrenal hyperplasia affects both sexes, it more often is recognized in female infants. It accounts for approximately 50 percent of all cases of ambiguous sexual differentiation. Despite its genetic origin, congenital adrenal hyperplasia is not associated with karyotypic abnormalities. The most typical abnormality of external genitalia is clitoral enlargement, which is usually accompanied by some degree of hypospadias and labioscrotal fusion.

3. **The answer is C.** *(Mattingly, ed 5. pp 33-36.)* The jack-knife position described in the question commonly gives rise to injury of the sciatic or peroneal nerve through the overstretching of the nerve over the sacrospinous ligament. The symptoms of footdrop and loss of sensation over the dorsal aspect of the foot classically accompany peroneal nerve injury. The ilioinguinal and genitofemoral nerves traverse the inguinal canal together with the round ligament. The obturator nerve, which runs along the lateral wall of the pelvis, can be damaged by deep retractors and during radical pelvic surgery. It supplies all of the adductor muscles of the thigh as well as provides the sensory supply to the medial aspects of the thigh. The internal pudendal nerve is derived from $S_2$-$S_3$ and supplies the vulva and perineum.

4. **The answer is E.** *(Sciarra, pp 8-9.)* The four portions of the fallopian tube in order from the ovary to the uterus are the infundibulum, a funnel-like dilatation; the ampulla; the narrow isthmus; and the interstitium, which opens into the uterine cavity at both cornua. The fallopian tube is usually 10 to 12 cm long, with the diameter of the lumen approximately 1 mm at the interstitial portion, 2.5 mm at the isthmus, 6 mm at the ampulla, and as much as 1 cm at the infundibular region. Both salpingitis and ectopic pregnancies occur most frequently in the ampullary region.

5. **The answer is A.** *(Mattingly, ed 5. pp 314-315.)* Habitual abortion is the most important indication for surgical treatment of women who have a double uterus. The abortion rate in women who have a double uterus is two to three times greater than that of the general population. Therefore, women who present with habitual abortion should be evaluated by hysterosalpingography to detect a possible double uterus. Dysmenorrhea, premature delivery, dyspareunia, and menometrorrhagia are other, less important indications for surgical intervention.

6. **The answer is A (1, 2, 3).** *(Thompson, ed 3. 148-150, 159-161, 348.)* Individuals who are carriers of a balanced D/G translocation have 45 chromosomes in each cell; one D-group and one G-group chromosome have fused, forming a chromosome that resembles a member of the C group. The risk for giving birth to children who have translocation Down's syndrome is substantially higher if the wife is the carrier (10 to 12 percent) than if the husband is the carrier (2 to 3 percent). Amniocentesis can determine whether the offspring will be unaffected, will carry the translocation, or will have the disease. Because a D/G translocation can be inherited from a parent (approximately 50 percent are familial), chromosome studies of family members are recommended.

7. **The answer is A (1, 2, 3).** *(Yen, pp 274-276.)* Individuals with a 45,X karyotype have Turner's syndrome (gonadal dysgenesis), a disorder in phenotypic females characterized by a variety of physical abnormalities. In addition to those listed in the question, pigmented nevi, a short fourth metacarpal, wide-set nipples, and renal and cardiovascular anomalies are common. Lymphedema presents as puffiness of the hands and feet at birth. Diabetes mellitus is also prevalent among these children. Gonadal dysgenesis, unlike other chromosomal abnormalities, is not related to maternal age.

8. **The answer is D (4).** *(Burrow, pp 820, 859.)* If a woman who has phenylketonuria, which is an autosomal recessive disorder, marries a carrier for this disease, the chance that offspring will be affected is 50 percent. Although phenylketonuria cannot be detected prenatally, screening of newborns and early institu-

tion of low-phenylalanine diets have made it possible for affected individuals to reach adulthood. It has become apparent that a high frequency of mental retardation exists in children of mothers who have phenylketonuria, even if these children do not themselves have the disease. Retardation in these children presumably is related to intrauterine exposure to high phenylalanine levels in the maternal blood.

**9. The answer is A (1, 2, 3).** *(Speroff, ed 2. p 245.)* Although monosomy of the X chromosome (45,XO) is the most common karyotype of patients who have Turner's syndrome, a variety of structural abnormalities of the X chromosome in addition to mosaics may be found in patients who have this disorder. Comparison of chromosomal abnormalities and phenotypic features in individuals who have gonadal dysgenesis indicates that the short stature and other clinical findings of the Turner's phenotype are associated with loss of the short arm of one X chromosome. Of the karyotypes listed in the question, all involve monosomy for a portion of the short arm of the X chromosome except 46,X,i(Xp). Individuals who have this karyotype have only one normal X chromosome; their other X chromosome, composed of a duplication of the normal short arm, is called an isochromosome. In essence, they are monosomic for the long arm of the X and trisomic for the short arm. This karyotype is associated with gonadal dysgenesis but not with the phenotypic features characteristic of individuals who have Turner's syndrome.

**10. The answer is B (1, 3).** *(Mattingly, ed 5. pp 165-166.)* Benefits of a low transverse abdominal incision are a decreased incidence of incisional hernias and cosmetic placement of the scar near the edge of the pubic hairline. The use of light anesthesia is contraindicated because it provides poor muscle relaxation. Bowel surgery is best approached with a vertical incision, especially if a colostomy is anticipated.

**11. The answer is A (1, 2, 3).** *(Parsons, ed 2. pp 683-686.)* Failure of fusion of the müllerian ducts can give rise to several types of uterine anomalies of which uterus bicornis unicollis is a representative type. This condition is associated with higher obstetrical complications, such as an increase in the rate of second trimester abortion and premature labor. If the pregnancies go to term, malpresentations such as breech and transverse lies are frequent. Also, prolonged labor, which is probably due to inadequate muscle development in the uterus; increased bleeding; and a higher incidence of fetal anomalies caused by defective implantation of the placenta, all occur far more commonly than in normal pregnancies. An intravenous pyelogram is mandatory in the workup of patients with uterine anomalies as there is an associated higher incidence of urinary tract anomalies. In uterus bicornis unicollis, there is a single cervix with a normal vagina.

12. **The answer is C (2, 4).** *(Parsons, ed 2. p 1606.)* An important feature of the lymphatic drainage of the vulva is the existence of drainage across the midline. The vulva drains first into the superficial inguinal lymph nodes, then into the deep femoral nodes, and finally into the external iliac lymph nodes. The clinical significance of this sequence for patients with carcinoma of the vulva is that the iliac nodes are probably free of the disease if the deep femoral nodes are not involved. Unlike the lymphatic drainage from the rest of the vulva, the drainage from the clitoral region bypasses the superficial inguinal nodes and passes directly to the deep femoral nodes. Thus, while the superficial nodes will usually also have metastases when the deep femoral nodes are implicated, it is possible for only the deep nodes to be involved if the carcinoma is in the midline near the clitoris.

13. **The answer is C (2, 4).** *(Pritchard, ed 16. pp 577, 1000.)* An infant with Potter's syndrome generally presents as a breech. After birth, the baby never is able to ventilate adequately. These infants rarely survive more than a few hours. The primary lesion in Potter's syndrome is thought to be renal. Because of renal agenesis, urine output is impossible, and oligohydramnios results. Oligohydramnios is believed to lead to pulmonary hypoplasia, because lack of amniotic fluid somehow restricts normal lung development. The characteristic facial anomalies (large, low-set ears and flattened nose) are thought to be related to pressure on the face increased by a lack of cushioning amniotic fluid. The diagnosis of Potter's syndrome has been made antenatally with the aid of ultrasonography. Demonstration of a fetal bladder that fills and empties should rule out Potter's syndrome. The absence of evidence of a bladder, despite repeated ultrasonographic examinations, would be compatible with the diagnosis. Amnion nodosum, another common finding in Potter's syndrome, consists of multiple opaque nodules in the amnion. Their etiology is not clear, but they represent fetal squames that have become "parasitic" on the membranes.

14. **The answer is B (1, 3).** *(Burrow, pp 416-433.)* Rubella syndrome in the newborn secondary to rubella infection during pregnancy (especially, but not exclusively, during the first trimester) is well known. Although cytomegalovirus infection is less familiar, it is thought to cause congenital anomalies in about 5000 newborns every year in the United States. The abnormalities are usually in the central nervous system and include microcephaly, cerebral calcifications, deafness, and other mental and motor disabilities. Although there have been some suggestions that influenza epidemics have led to a subsequent rise in the incidence of childhood leukemia, this relationship has not been established; in fact, there is no proof that influenza is associated with any anomalies. Mumps is relatively common during pregnancy, but prospective studies have failed to show any associated congenital anomalies.

Anatomy, Genetics, and Embryology 13

**15-19. The answers are: 15-D, 16-A, 17-B, 18-E, 19-C.** *(Mattingly, ed 5. pp 36-38.)* The blood supply of the pelvic organs and musculature is derived primarily from the hypogastric artery. The uterine artery arises from the anterior division of the hypogastric artery and supplies the vagina, uterus, and fallopian tubes. The bladder is also supplied by the vesical branches of the hypogastric artery, which terminates as the internal pudendal artery supplying the perineum, labia, and clitoris, as well as the thigh muscles. The uterine veins, which drain into the internal iliac veins, generally follow the course of the uterine arteries. Together, they course superiorly to the ureters along the base of the broad ligaments.

The two ovarian veins follow different courses. The right ovarian vein drains into the inferior vena cava just below the level of the right renal vein, while the left ovarian vein drains into the left renal vein. The right ovarian vein may become distended during pregnancy, causing partial obstruction of the ureter proximal to its course. This has been postulated to be a cause of right hydronephrosis in pregnancy. The ovarian artery arises from the abdominal aorta. It courses through the infundibulopelvic ligament and supplies the ovary and the fallopian tube.

A thorough understanding of the above-mentioned relationships is essential in gynecological surgery, especially in cases of hemorrhage requiring hypogastric artery ligation.

**20-24. The answers are: 20-D, 21-B, 22-A, 23-C, 24-E.** *(Blaustein, pp 9-11. Green, ed 3. pp 77-80, 88-96, 103, 109.)* In the female, the urethral folds give rise to the labia minora, while the labia majora are formed from the genital swellings. It is believed that the development of external genitalia is dependent on the presence of hormones during the intrauterine period. With the absence of androgens and the inducer substance in females, the wolffian duct system regresses while the external genitalia develop under the influence of estrogen from both maternal and placental sources.

In the male, the genital tubercle gives rise to the phallus, while in the female it elongates minimally to form the clitoris. Clitoral hypertrophy can occur in conditions where there is an abnormally high level of circulating androgens during the critical phase of development of the external genitalia. Congenital adrenal hyperplasia and mixed gonadal dysgenesis are two clinical situations that may present with clitoral hypertrophy.

There are several theories to explain the embryological origin of the vagina; however, it is generally accepted that the upper two-thirds of the vagina are of müllerian duct origin while the lower one-third is of urogenital sinus origin, which seems to explain in part the congenital anomalies that arise in this anatomical region. A common anomaly of urogenital sinus origin is imperforate hymen, which is easily treated by hymenotomy. Congenital absence of the vagina is an anomaly of müllerian duct origin and, as such, usually involves an absence of only the upper two-thirds of the vagina, as well as an absence of the uterus and fallopian tubes in most cases.

In the female, the müllerian ducts give rise to the fallopian tubes, uterus, and cervix. Imperfect fusion of the müllerian ducts can give rise to a whole spectrum of uterine anomalies, which may be associated with clinical entities like habitual abortions, prematurity, and fetal malpositions. Patients with proven müllerian duct anomalies should have an intravenous pyelogram to rule out urinary tract anomalies that may be present.

**25-29. The answers are: 25-B, 26-C, 27-A, 28-D, 29-E.** *(Blaustein, pp 9-10, 70. Novak, ed 9. pp 1-3, 438.)* The male homologue of the round ligament is the gubernaculum testis. It is a cordlike structure extending from the lower pole of the testis to the scrotum. Abnormalities of this structure are associated with maldescent of the testes. The round ligaments play a minor role in support of the uterus.

The prostate gland corresponds with the paraurethral glands in females. Clinically, these glands and their canals, which open into both the urethra and the Skene's ducts, can serve as a reservoir for gonococcal infections. Also, these glands can become cystic with chronic infections, giving rise to suburethral diverticula.

In the embryological development of the external genitalia of the female, the urethral folds and the genital swellings do **not** fuse, giving rise to the labia minora and the labia majora, respectively. The contrary is true in the male, as the urethral folds fuse to form the penis, while the scrotum is formed by the fusion of the genital swellings.

The vas deferens and Gartner's duct are both derived from the wolffian-duct system. Cysts of Gartner's duct, when present, are usually found along the anterolateral wall of the vagina. They are usually asymptomatic and rarely require surgical intervention.

Embryologically, the male phallus and the female clitoris both arise from the genital tubercle. Hypertrophy of the clitoris can occur if there is a high level of androgens present during the early development of the external genitalia.

**30-34. The answers are: 30-D, 31-E, 32-B, 33-A, 34-E.** *(Burrow, pp 817, 832, 842-843, 852, 855-859, 861.)* Huntington's chorea is an autosomal dominant disorder causing progressive mental deterioration and eventual dementia. It has its clinical onset during the late reproductive years or following the reproductive years. The chance that the woman described in the question has inherited the gene from her father is 1:2. Therefore, the chance that her child will inherit the disease is 25 percent ($1/2 \times 1/2 = 1/4$).

The frequency of Tay-Sachs disease is markedly higher among American Jews of Ashkenazi descent than in the general United States population. Screen-

## Anatomy, Genetics, and Embryology 15

ing studies indicate that the carrier frequency for the Tay-Sachs gene in this ethnic group is approximately 1:30, making the incidence of the disease 1:3600 (1/30 x 1/30 x 1/4). Carrier testing and prenatal diagnosis can help detect the presence of the disease in a fetus and therefore provide a basis for deciding whether or not to continue the pregnancy.

Although the recurrence rate for trisomy 21 (Down's syndrome) is not well defined, it generally is stated to be 1 percent. This figure is based on documented recurrences in families in which one parent has a low-percentage mosaicism for a cell line with a 47,XX,+21 or 47,XY,+21 chromosome constitution. In one series of prenatal diagnoses, five trisomic fetuses were discovered in 485 pregnancies examined for Down's syndrome. The risk for having a child with Down's syndrome is not known to be increased in other relatives of children who have a primary trisomy (47,XX,+21 or 47,XY,+21). When a patient has a family history of Down's syndrome, chromosome analysis should be performed to determine if the disease is a sporadic event (primary trisomy) or a translocation. If the affected family member has translocation Down's syndrome, a chromosome study of that child's parents, relatives, or both is indicated to ascertain whether the translocation is familial or a mutation.

Neural tube defects follow a multifactorial mode of inheritance. When there have been sufficient data for the derivation of empiric risk figures, the risk for having a child with a neural tube defect has been found to increase with the birth of each affected child. The risk following the birth of one child with a neural tube defect is 3 to 5 percent; the risk following the birth of the second affected child is 12 to 13 percent. Prenatal diagnosis, based on the amniotic fluid level of alpha-fetoprotein as well as on other adjunctive studies, is available.

# Puberty, Menstruation, Menopause, Sexuality, and Conception

**DIRECTIONS:** Each question below contains five suggested answers. Choose the one **best** response to each question.

35. In the testis, which of the following can be **directly** influenced by luteinizing hormone (LH)?

(A) Leydig cells
(B) Sertoli cells
(C) Leydig cells and Sertoli cells
(D) Leydig cells and seminiferous tubules
(E) Sertoli cells and seminiferous tubules

36. What is the usual order of appearance of the signs of normal puberty?

(A) Axillary hair, breast buds, pubic hair, and menarche
(B) Breast buds, axillary hair, pubic hair, and menarche
(C) Breast buds, pubic hair, axillary hair, and menarche
(D) Pubic hair, menarche, breast buds, and axillary hair
(E) Pubic hair, breast buds, menarche, and axillary hair

37. All of the following steps in the mechanism of action of adrenocorticotropic hormone (ACTH) are correct EXCEPT that

(A) ACTH is bound by specific surface receptors on the adrenal cortical cell
(B) in the presence of magnesium, adenylcyclase is activated and the intracellular concentration of adenosine $3':5'$-cyclic phosphate (cyclic AMP) increases
(C) cyclic AMP phosphorylates key enzymes
(D) key enzymes facilitate the conversion of cholesterol to pregnenolone
(E) synthesis of new proteins occurs and increases adrenal weight

38. The hormone primarily responsible for production of sex steroids is

(A) follicle-stimulating hormone (FSH)
(B) luteinizing hormone (LH)
(C) adrenocorticotropic hormone (ACTH)
(D) thyroid-stimulating hormone (TSH)
(E) prolactin

39. According to Masters and Johnson, factors that increase the likelihood of female orgasm during intercourse include

(A) a larger clitoral glans
(B) a clitoris located closer to the vaginal introitus
(C) erection of the clitoral shaft
(D) male superior coital position
(E) none of the above

40. All of the following phases or periods of the sex response cycle, as described by Masters and Johnson, are present in both men and women EXCEPT

(A) resolution
(B) excitement
(C) orgasmic
(D) refractory
(E) plateau

41. If a man received a severe thermal trauma to his testes, his previously normal sperm count would become depressed in about

(A)  1 day
(B)  7 days
(C)  30 days
(D)  75 days
(E)  100 days

42. If the aim of artificial insemination is to inseminate a woman at the time of ovulation, the best time for insemination, relative to the measured LH peak, is

(A) 12 to 24 hours before the LH peak
(B) at the peak
(C) 2 to 5 hours after the peak
(D) 16 to 24 hours after the peak
(E) 25 to 48 hours after the peak

43. Which of the following statements about the derivation of urinary testosterone in men is true?

(A) One hundred percent is testicular in origin
(B) Ninety-five percent is derived from the testes and five percent from the adrenal glands
(C) Fifty percent is derived from the testes and fifty percent from the adrenal glands
(D) One hundred percent is adrenal in origin
(E) Its derivation cannot be accurately determined

44. A patient with a 38-day ovulatory cycle who asks her physician when she is most likely to conceive should be told that ovulation would most probably occur on day

(A) 18
(B) 20
(C) 22
(D) 24
(E) 26

**DIRECTIONS:** Each question below contains four suggested answers of which **one** or **more** is correct. Choose the answer:

| A | if | 1, 2, and 3 | are correct |
|---|---|---|---|
| B | if | 1 and 3 | are correct |
| C | if | 2 and 4 | are correct |
| D | if | 4 | is correct |
| E | if | 1, 2, 3, and 4 | are correct |

45. The menopause invariably is accompanied by

(1) osteoporosis
(2) anxiety and depression
(3) cardiovascular degeneration
(4) decreased serum estrogen levels

46. The major estrogenic substances in postmenopausal women include

(1) estradiol
(2) estrone
(3) estriol
(4) androstenedione

47. Waning estrogen levels in perimenopausal women can produce which of the following responses?

(1) Vasomotor instability
(2) Atrophic vaginitis
(3) Decreased libido
(4) Osteoporosis

48. Rising estradiol levels can have which of the following hormonal effects?

(1) Suppression of LH
(2) Stimulation of LH
(3) Suppression of FSH
(4) Stimulation of FSH

49. The major pituitary hormones responsible for the luteal phases of the menstrual cycle include

(1) prolactin
(2) FSH
(3) LH
(4) growth hormone

50. The luteal phase of the menstrual cycle primarily involves

(1) the $\Delta^4$-3-ketone pathway
(2) the $\Delta^5$-3$\beta$-hydroxy pathway
(3) granulosa cells
(4) theca cells

51. Cholesterol can be synthesized from acetate by which of the following organs?

(1) Ovary
(2) Adrenal gland
(3) Testis
(4) Placenta

52. Physiological processes that are estrogen-dependent in women include which of the following?

(1) Menses
(2) Vaginal cornification
(3) Appearance of axillary hair
(4) Cervical mucus formation

53. Characteristics of the gonadotropins (FSH and LH) include
(1) stimulation of the production of primordial follicles
(2) stimulation of the production of estrogen by thecal cells
(3) stimulation of the production of spermatozoa and testosterone in men who have hypopituitarism
(4) a glycoprotein structure

54. Polypeptide structure and direct inducement of hormonal changes in target organs are characteristics of which of the following hormones?
(1) Prolactin
(2) Growth hormone
(3) Chorionic somatomammotropin
(4) Thyrotropin

55. True statements about sexual activity in late pregnancy include which of the following?
(1) Intercourse during the third trimester can lead to premature labor
(2) Intercourse during the third trimester can promote premature rupture of membranes and intrauterine infection
(3) Prostaglandins in semen have been shown to contribute to the initiation of labor
(4) Orgasm is contraindicated in women who have a history of premature labor

56. Physiological actions occurring during the plateau phase of sexual excitement in women include
(1) areolar tumescence
(2) systolic blood pressure elevations
(3) involuntary skeletal muscle contractions
(4) involuntary contractions of the rectal sphincter

57. Significant components of vaginal lubrication include
(1) fluid from Skene's glands
(2) mucus produced by endocervical glands
(3) viscous fluid from Bartholin's glands
(4) transudatelike material from the vaginal walls

58. The contraceptive effect of birth control pills containing both synthetic estrogen and progestin is related to the
(1) inhibition of ovulation
(2) impaired penetrability of sperm into the cervical mucus
(3) atrophic changes of the endometrium impairing implantation
(4) uterotubal hypermotility impairing sperm transport

**DIRECTIONS:** The group of questions below consists of lettered choices followed by several numbered items. For each numbered item select the **one** lettered choice with which it is **most** closely associated. Each lettered choice may be used once, more than once, or not at all.

**Questions 59-63**

Match each action listed below with the appropriate enzyme.

(A) Adenylcyclase
(B) 5α-Reductase
(C) 17β-Hydroxylase
(D) 20-Hydroxylase
(E) 21-Dehydroxylase

59. Is activated by LH

60. Converts androstenedione to testosterone

61. Converts testosterone to dihydrotestosterone

62. Catalyzes the first step in the production of hormonal steroids from cholesterol

63. Causes massive adrenal enlargement when congenitally deficient, is associated with poor survival of the affected infants, and can lead to the formation of female genitalia in genotypically male infants

# Puberty, Menstruation, Menopause, Sexuality, and Conception
# Answers

**35. The answer is A.** *(Williams, ed 5. pp 324-329.)* In the testis, Leydig cells produce testosterone, Sertoli cells primarily provide structural support and nutrition, and seminiferous tubules produce sperm. Leydig cells are under the influence of luteinizing hormone (LH) in a negative-feedback relationship. Testosterone produced by Leydig cells regulates spermatogenesis; therefore, seminiferous tubules are indirectly affected by LH secretion.

**36. The answer is C.** *(Speroff, ed 2. p 253.)* The appearance of breast buds is dependent on early estrogen production and is usually the first sign of puberty. Increased production of androgens causes the development of pubic hair and, about 2 years later, axillary hair. Menarche then occurs, usually after the growth spurt has peaked.

**37. The answer is B.** *(Williams, ed 5. p 38.)* Adrenocorticotropic hormone (ACTH) binds to specific cell-surface receptors in the adrenal cortex and is concentrated from the plasma. The combined action of ACTH and calcium stimulates adenylcyclase to catalyze production of adenosine $3':5'$-cyclic phosphate (cyclic AMP), which in turn causes enzyme phosphorylation. These enzymes convert precursors to active hormones; cholesterol, for example, is converted enzymatically to pregnenolone. Cyclic AMP also induces synthesis of RNA, which in turn stimulates protein synthesis; as a result, adrenal weight is increased.

**38. The answer is B.** *(Speroff, ed 2. pp 7-10.)* Follicle-stimulating hormone (FSH) is responsible for spermatocyte production and ovum maturation, and luteinizing hormone (LH) is primarily responsible for production of hormones (e.g., the production of progesterone by the granulosa cells of the ovary). Prolactin, adrenocorticotropic hormone (ACTH), and thyroid-stimulating hormone (TSH) have no known role in sex-steroid production. LH probably is responsible for the actual act of ovulation and may activate cholesterol esterase, which catalyzes production of cholesterol (the precursor of steroids and, therefore, of the sex steroids) and free fatty acids (prostaglandin precursors).

**39. The answer is E.** *(Dickinson, p 46. Dickinson, JAMA 85:1113-1117, 1925. Masters, 1966. pp 48, 56-59.)* Masters and Johnson have shown that the size of the clitoris bears no relation to increased orgasmic capacity. Similarly, the distance between the clitoris and the vaginal introitus makes little difference, because clitoral stimulation during coition is provided largely by traction on the clitoral hood via the labia minora, which are moved during penile thrusting. Direct clitoral stimulation can be achieved only by the lateral and female superior coital positions. Erection of the clitoris is likewise not related to orgasmic capacity. Masters and Johnson's findings agree with those of earlier researchers, including Dickinson and Pierson.

**40. The answer is D.** *(Masters, 1966. pp 4-7, 13.)* Masters and Johnson observed the sexual responses of 382 women and 312 men. They arbitrarily divided the sex response cycle of men and women into the excitement phase, the plateau phase, the orgasmic phase, and the resolution phase. After orgasm, men, but not women, must wait until a refractory period has passed before effective restimulation is possible. The length of this refractory period increases with age.

**41. The answer is D.** *(Speroff, ed 2. p 365.)* Severe thermal trauma to the testes, such as that caused by extremes of cold or heat, can inhibit the development of sperm. Depression in the sperm count usually appears in about 75 days, the length of time in which an immature spermatid develops into a spermatozoon. Either oligospermia or azoospermia can result.

**42. The answer is D.** *(Speroff, ed 2. pp 57, 371.)* Because ovulation occurs 16 to 24 hours after the LH peak, this is the best time to artificially inseminate a woman. An ovum can be fertilized at any time during the first 12 hours after ovulation. The fertile life of sperm within the female genital tract is not known precisely, but it has been estimated to be 24 to 48 hours. In practice, artificial insemination is performed 1 or 2 days before the rise of basal body temperature, which indicates approximately the time of ovulation.

**43. The answer is B.** *(Williams, ed 5. p 237. Yen, p 114.)* In man, testosterone is produced by the testes and the adrenal glands. The Leydig cells in the testes are the primary sites for testosterone production, with the first step involving the synthesis of cholesterol from acetate, followed by the cleavage of the cholesterol side chain, giving rise to pregnenolone, which is the main precursor for steroid synthesis in the testes. Ninety-five percent of testosterone is derived in this manner. The adrenal glands account for the remaining 5 percent of testosterone production through the transformation of $\Delta^4$-androstenedione to testosterone glucuronide, principally in the liver.

**44. The answer is D.** *(Pritchard, ed 16. p 49. Speroff, ed 2. p 58.)* Although the time of ovulation may vary, it is well accepted that it usually occurs approximately 14 days before the onset of the next menstrual period. This reflects the constant luteal phase of the menstrual cycle. The follicular phase in women, which encompasses the period of both follicular maturation and growth, is responsible for the variability in cycle length among different women. For this reason, the rhythm method of family planning has a poor use-effectiveness record among women with irregular menstrual cycles.

**45. The answer is D (4).** *(Gilman, ed 6. p 1426. Wynn, ed 2. pp 217-218.)* The *sine qua non* of the menopause is ovarian failure; a marked decrease in estrogen production subsequently results, and a secondary increase in the production of FSH by the pituitary is noted. Symptoms of emotional upset may be due more to a change in life situation than to a change in hormonal balance. Cardiovascular and bony degeneration occurs in some, but by no means all, women. Estrogen replacement therapy should probably be limited to women with climacteric symptoms because recent data suggest that estrogen use by postmenopausal women may be associated with the development of endometrial carcinoma; its use is least effective in treating women who develop osteoporosis.

**46. The answer is C (2, 4).** *(Green, ed 3. p 567. Speroff, ed 2. pp 74-78.)* During their reproductive years, the major estrogenic substance produced by women is estradiol. Pregnancy brings about an enormous rise in the level of estriol. With the cessation of ovulation, estradiol production falls, and production of estrone and androstenedione increases. Androstenedione is converted peripherally in adipose tissue to estrone, which may be sufficient to maintain estrogen dependent tissues in some women in the early postmenopausal period. With advancing age, the precursors for estrogen production provided by the adrenals will eventually prove inadequate, and this withdrawal of estrogen can result in psychological mood changes, venomotor instability, and atrophic conditions.

**47. The answer is E (all).** *(Speroff, ed 2. pp 77-82.)* In menopausal and postmenopausal women, waning estrogen levels can produce atrophic vaginitis, decreased libido, vasomotor instability, osteoporosis, and psychological symptoms (including depression and anxiety). Vasomotor instability causes the familiar hot flashes of menopausal women. These responses may be due to an unstable relationship, caused by decreased estrogen levels, between the autonomic nervous system and the hypothalamus.

**48. The answer is A (1, 2, 3).** *(Speroff, ed 2. pp 52-53.)* Estradiol has a negative-feedback relationship with FSH and both a negative-feedback and a positive-feedback relationship with LH. Rising estradiol levels suppress the production of FSH and LH. As estradiol levels continue to increase, however, LH levels begin to rise. Negative feedback (suppression of LH and FSH production) is mediated by estradiol effects on the hypothalamus and pituitary gland; positive feedback (increase in LH) also is controlled by hypothalamic centers.

**49. The answer is B (1, 3).** *(Green, ed 3. p 148.)* In the early part of the menstrual cycle, FSH seems to be the hormone responsible in large part for maturation of ovarian follicles. At midcycle there is a surge of LH, and high levels are sustained throughout the luteal phase. Secretion of prolactin, which probably aids in the luteinization of the follicle, also occurs at this time.

**50. The answer is B (1, 3).** *(Speroff, ed 2. pp 9-10.)* In the luteal phase of the menstrual cycle, granulosa cells produce estrogen by way of the $\Delta^4$-3-ketone pathway, in which progesterone is a precursor. Theca cells in the follicular phase of the menstrual cycle manufacture estrogen by the $\Delta^5$-3$\beta$-hydroxy pathway; pregnenolone, dehydroepiandrosterone, and estradiol—but not progesterone—are essential precursors of this pathway.

**51. The answer is A (1, 2, 3).** *(Speroff, ed 2. p 7.)* The conversion of acetate to cholesterol and, hence, to all the other steroid hormones can occur in the ovary, testis, and adrenal gland. The placenta, however, lacks the essential enzyme systems to perform this synthesis. Therefore, cholesterol, the basic building block in the synthesis of steroid hormones, must be supplied to the placenta. The fetus and the mother supply the cholesterol essential for steroidogenesis in the placenta. It has been suggested that the maternal cholesterol serves as the precursor for progesterone production, while fetal cholesterol is used for estrogen production.

**52. The answer is E (all).** *(Speroff, ed 2. p 45.)* The presence of estrogen in a pubertal woman stimulates the formation of secondary sex characteristics, including development of breasts, appearance of axillary hair, production of cervical mucus, and vaginal cornification. As estrogen levels increase, menses begins and ovulation is maintained for several decades. Decreasing levels of estrogen lower the frequency of ovulation, eventually leading to the menopause.

**53. The answer is E (all).** *(Williams, ed 5. pp 41-44.)* The gonadotropins (FSH and LH) are glycoproteins. In women, they stimulate the production of one or more primordial follicles and induce thecal cells in the ovary to produce estro-

Puberty, Menstruation, and Menopause    25

gen. In a man who has hypopituitarism, the gonadotropins can cause production of spermatozoa and testosterone.

**54. The answer is A (1, 2, 3).** *(Williams, ed 5. p 46.)* Growth hormone and chorionic somatomammotropin are polypeptide hormones composed of 191 amino-acid subunits, of which 161 are identical (the other 30 are closely related and vary by only a simple base change in the DNA template). Although the structure of human prolactin is not yet clearly established, it too is a polypeptide hormone of close to 200 subunits, many of which are in the same sequence as the other two hormones. Prolactin, growth hormone, and chorionic somatomammotropin all are able to induce hormonal changes directly in their target organs. Thyrotropin is a glycoprotein; its only physiological action is stimulation of the thyroid gland to produce another hormone, thyroxine, which is the mediator of thyroid activity.

**55. The answer is D (4).** *(Green, ed 2. pp 177-189.)* Several clinical surveys have failed to reveal any firm association between intercourse and premature labor, premature rupture of membranes, or intrauterine infection. On the other hand, orgasm, regardless of how it is achieved, can be harmful to women who have a history of premature delivery or a prematurely ripe cervix, because of accompanying uterine contractions. A fetal head that is engaged in the pelvis may be bumped during coitus; although this may frighten the parents, no demonstrable harm to the infant results. The physiological role of prostaglandins in human semen is unknown.

**56. The answer is A (1, 2, 3).** *(Masters, 1966. pp 27-37.)* The response of women to sexual stimulation is generalized and affects many different organ systems. Physiological responses include superficial and deep vasocongestion accounting for, among other things, enlargement and changes of color of extragenital and genital areas. Voluntary and involuntary myotonia, both generalized and specific, also may occur, although involuntary contractions of the rectal sphincter are usually detected only during the orgasmic phase.

**57. The answer is D (4).** *(Masters, 1966. p 69.)* Masters and Johnson observed a transudatelike fluid emanating directly from the vaginal walls during sexual response. This mucoid material, which is sufficient for complete vaginal lubrication, is produced by transudation from the venous plexus surrounding the vagina and appears seconds after the initiation of sexual excitement. No activity by Skene's glands was noted, and production of cervical mucus during sexual stimulation was observed in only a very few subjects. Fluid from Bartholin's glands appears long after vaginal lubrication is well established; it may, however, make a minor contribution to lubrication in the late plateau phase.

**58. The answer is A (1, 2, 3).** *(Wynn, ed 2. p 232.)* The marked effectiveness of the combined oral contraceptive pill, which contains a synthetic estrogen and a progestin, is related to its multiple antifertility actions. The primary effect is to suppress gonadotropins, thus inhibiting ovulation. The prolonged progestational effect also causes thickening of the cervical mucus and atrophic changes of the endometrium, thus impairing sperm penetrability and ovum implantation, respectively.

**59-63. The answers are: 59-A, 60-C, 61-B, 62-D, 63-D.** *(Williams, ed 5. pp 276, 325, 330-332.)* Testosterone reaching a target organ, such as the prostate gland, is converted to dihydrotestosterone by 5α-reductase, an enzyme in the cell wall or cell membrane. Adenylcyclase, which is an intracellular enzyme activated by the presence of LH, catalyzes the formation of cyclic AMP, which then activates other intracellular enzyme reactions. The enzyme 17β-hydroxylase is found primarily in the testis but also in the adrenal gland; it converts androstenedione to testosterone by hydroxylating the 17 position.

The conversion of cholesterol into steroid hormones begins with hydroxylation at the 20 position followed by cleavage of the six-carbon side chain (carbons 22 to 27); both reactions, which result in production of pregnenolone, are catalyzed by 20-hydroxylase (also known as cholesterol desmolase). Congenital deficiencies of this enzyme can cause the adrenal glands to fill with cholesterol and become greatly enlarged; affected infants, some of whom may be phenotypic females but genotypic males, have a poor prognosis.

# Pregnancy, Lactation, and Puerperium

**DIRECTIONS**: Each question below contains five suggested answers. Choose the **one best** response to each question.

64. An elevation of prolactin levels is caused by all of the following physiological states EXCEPT

(A) sleep
(B) stress
(C) exercise
(D) parturition
(E) puerperium

65. In a normal pregnancy, the maximum amniotic fluid volume is approximately

(A) 800 ml
(B) 1000 ml
(C) 1200 ml
(D) 1400 ml
(E) 1600 ml

66. The maternal mortality rate refers to the number of maternal deaths that occur as the result of the reproductive process per

(A) 1000 births
(B) 10,000 births
(C) 100,000 births
(D) 10,000 live births
(E) 100,000 live births

67. The maximum amniotic fluid volume is usually reached at what gestational age?

(A) 32 to 34 weeks
(B) 34 to 36 weeks
(C) 36 to 38 weeks
(D) 38 to 40 weeks
(E) 40 to 42 weeks

68. All of the following statements about the endometrial Arias-Stella reaction in pregnant women are true EXCEPT that

(A) it was first described in association with tubal pregnancy
(B) it is a reaction of glandular epithelial cells
(C) it is a sign of impending fetal death
(D) affected cells have abundant, eosinophilic-staining cytoplasm
(E) the nuclei of affected cells are hyperchromatic and increased in size

69. At 12 weeks gestation, amniotic fluid volume is approximately

(A) 50 ml
(B) 100 ml
(C) 150 ml
(D) 200 ml
(E) 250 ml

70. During pregnancy a woman needs additional iron to satisfy the demands of the fetus, the placenta, and her own increasing hemoglobin mass. The total antepartum iron need is approximately

(A) 250 mg
(B) 800 mg
(C) 1350 mg
(D) 1900 mg
(E) none of the above

71. As pregnancy progresses, which of the following hematological changes occurs?

(A) Plasma volume increases proportionally more than red-cell volume
(B) Red-cell volume increases proportionally more than plasma volume
(C) Plasma volume increases and red-cell volume remains constant
(D) Red-cell volume decreases and plasma volume remains constant
(E) Neither plasma volume nor red-cell volume changes

72. Clinical studies have demonstrated which of the following blood pressure changes in the second trimester of pregnancy as compared with the beginning of pregnancy?

(A) Significantly reduced systolic and diastolic blood pressures
(B) Reduced systolic blood pressure and relatively unchanged diastolic blood pressure
(C) Relatively unchanged systolic blood pressure and reduced diastolic blood pressure
(D) Increased systolic blood pressure and relatively unchanged diastolic blood pressure
(E) Significantly increased systolic and diastolic blood pressures

73. All of the following statements about renal function in normal pregnancy are true EXCEPT that

(A) caliceal, renal pelvic, and ureteral dilatation can occur as early as the second trimester
(B) hormonal and mechanical factors have been implicated as causes of ureteral dilatation in the third trimester
(C) glomerular filtration rate increases about 50 percent over values in nonpregnant women
(D) renal plasma flow increases about 35 percent over values in nonpregnant women
(E) creatinine clearance is an accurate reflection of glomerular filtration rate during pregnancy

74. Which of the following statements best characterizes the estrogen present in maternal urine?

(A) Its concentration is decreased during pregnancy
(B) It is 80 to 85 percent estriol at term
(C) It is 50 percent estradiol at term
(D) Its excretion is normal at term in patients who have placental sulfatase deficiency
(E) Its excretion is unrelated to fetal adrenal or hepatic function

75. During the first postpartum week, the uterus will lose what percent of its immediate postpartum weight?

(A) 10 percent
(B) 30 percent
(C) 50 percent
(D) 70 percent
(E) 90 percent

76. A 23-year-old woman (gravida 2, para 2) calls her physician 7 days postpartum because she is concerned that she is still bleeding from the vagina. It would be appropriate to tell this woman that it is normal for bloody lochia to last up to

(A) 2 days
(B) 5 days
(C) 8 days
(D) 11 days
(E) 14 days

**DIRECTIONS**: Each question below contains four suggested answers of which **one** or **more** is correct. Choose the answer:

| | | | |
|---|---|---|---|
| A | if | 1, 2, and 3 | are correct |
| B | if | 1 and 3 | are correct |
| C | if | 2 and 4 | are correct |
| D | if | 4 | is correct |
| E | if | 1, 2, 3, and 4 | are correct |

77. The physiological effects of endogenous oxytocin include

(1) relaxation of vascular smooth muscles
(2) initiation of milk production
(3) a marked antidiuretic-hormone effect
(4) stimulation of uterine contractions

78. True statements about postpartum lactation include which of the following?

(1) Breast engorgement occurs during the first postpartum day
(2) Only colostrum is produced at the time of delivery
(3) Prolactin levels rise steadily after delivery and peak at 1 month postpartum
(4) Oxytocin is not crucial for the production of milk

79. Which of the following laboratory values can be expected to increase during pregnancy?

(1) Serum albumin
(2) Plasma fibrinogen
(3) Blood urea nitrogen
(4) Erythrocyte sedimentation rate

80. Urinary estriol levels can decrease in women taking

(1) methenamine mandelate (Mandelamine)
(2) ampicillin
(3) corticosteroids
(4) phenolphthalein cathartics

81. Which of the following physiological changes can occur during a normal pregnancy?

(1) Decrease in fasting blood $\beta$-hydroxybutyric acid
(2) Increase in postprandial blood glucose
(3) Increase in fasting blood glucose
(4) Increase in postprandial insulin

82. Pregnancy can be considered diabetogenic because elevated levels of which of the following substances increase insulin secretion?

(1) Progesterone
(2) Estrogen
(3) Growth hormone
(4) Human chorionic sommatomammotropin

83. Which of the following thyroxine-related changes can occur during pregnancy?
(1) Increase of total serum thyroxine
(2) Increase of free thyroxine
(3) Increase of thyroxine-binding globulin
(4) Decrease of thyroid-stimulating hormone

84. Prolactin secretion is inhibited by which of the following compounds?
(1) Phenothiazines
(2) Alpha-methyldopa
(3) Serotonin
(4) Levodopa

85. In the mother, suckling leads to which of the following responses?
(1) Release of oxytocin
(2) Decrease of prolactin inhibitory factor
(3) Decrease of hypothalamic dopamine
(4) Increase of luteinizing-hormone releasing factor

# Pregnancy, Lactation, and Puerperium

## Answers

**64. The answer is E.** *(Yen, pp 158-165.)* Prolactin is released episodically in humans, with the highest levels being recorded during the nocturnal sleeping hours and the lowest levels during the waking hours of 10 A.M. to 12 P.M. Several other physiological stimuli, such as the stress of anesthesia, surgery, and exercise, have been shown to cause a rise in prolactin levels. In women, prolactin levels start to rise during the first trimester of pregnancy to a concentration ten times greater than that of the nonpregnant state. In the puerperium, prolactin levels decrease, reaching the normal range by the second or third week after delivery.

**65. The answer is B.** *(Pritchard, ed 16. pp 578-582.)* In a normal pregnancy, the maximum amniotic fluid volume is approximately 100 ml (1 L). When this volume is reached, the uterus may still be indented, and the fetal parts may be readily palpated. It is important to appreciate the normal volume of amniotic fluid in order to make an early clinical diagnosis of developing oligohydramnios (< 30 ml of amniotic fluid) or polyhydramnios (> 2000 ml of amniotic fluid). Oligohydramnios may lead to fetal deformities and pulmonary hypoplasia, while polyhydramnios greatly increases the incidence of fetal malformation and perinatal mortality owing to premature birth.

**66. The answer is E.** *(Pritchard, ed 16. p 3.)* The maternal mortality rate is calculated per 100,000 live births. Although there have been marked advances in prenatal care associated with a declining maternal mortality rate over the past 25 years, there still exist subgroups of the female population at much higher risk. These include black women (apparently because of social and economic conditions), women of high parity, and the older gravida. About 50 percent of maternal deaths in the United States are caused by hemorrhage, hypertension, or infection.

**67. The answer is C.** *(Pritchard, ed 16. pp 206-208.)* The maximum amniotic fluid volume of 1 L is reached at 36 to 38 weeks gestation. A decrease in volume is usually noted as term approaches, and in the post-term pregnancy clinically apparent oligohydramnios may develop. Oligohydramnios may also occur in association with fetal renal agenesis (Potter's syndrome) and in some cases of intrauterine growth retardation.

**68. The answer is C.** *(Mattingly, ed 5. p 372.)* Although the Arias-Stella reaction was first described in association with tubal pregnancy, it can occur in association with any condition in which active chorial tissue is present; these conditions include abortions, syncytial endometritis, hydatidiform mole, and choriocarcinoma. The Arias-Stella reaction affects glandular epithelial cells of the endometrium. These cells have abundant, vacuolated, eosinophilic cytoplasm and enlarged, hyperchromatic nuclei. This endometrial-gland reaction occurs after fetal death.

**69. The answer is A.** *(Pritchard, ed 16. pp 206, 603.)* At 12 weeks gestation, amniotic fluid volume is approximately 50 ml, rapidly increasing to about 200 ml by 16 weeks. For this reason, pregnancy termination by intra-amniotic instillation of saline or prostaglandin solutions is extremely difficult at 12 weeks but becomes relatively simple beyond 16 weeks. Some authorities believe that termination by suction abortion is dangerous beyond 12 weeks, and that the month between 12 and 16 weeks is a time when no method is safe. More recently, however, several studies have indicated that surgical abortion through the vagina is safe up to at least 16 weeks gestation.

**70. The answer is B.** *(Pritchard, ed 16. pp 234-235.)* The fetus and placenta contain approximately 300 mg of elemental iron at birth. In addition, the maternal increase in hemoglobin mass accounts for about 500 mg of elemental iron. Thus, the total antepartum iron requirement is 800 mg. Most of this iron is needed during the second half of pregnancy, at an approximate rate of 5.7 mg daily during the last 140 days. However, because about 1 mg of iron is excreted daily, the total daily iron need is almost 7 mg during the second half of pregnancy. Most women of childbearing age cannot mobilize this much iron, and supplemental iron must be given to prevent iron deficiency. The usual iron supplement, ferrous sulfate, contains 20 percent elemental iron. Thus, a 325 mg tablet contains about 65 mg of elemental iron, of which 10 to 20 percent will be absorbed. Most prenatal vitamins contain 60 or 65 mg of iron, and these should be adequate for a healthy pregnant woman. If iron stores have been depleted by poor dietary habits, recent childbirth, or other causes, however, additional iron supplementation may be necessary.

**71. The answer is A.** *(Peck, Clin Obstet Gynecol 22:785-789, 1979.)* During pregnancy, the plasma volume increases by about 40 percent and the red-cell volume increases by about 30 percent. The rapid increase in the plasma volume occurs during early pregnancy, while the red-cell volume rises more rapidly after the first trimester of pregnancy. As a result, the hematocrit during the first trimester and most of the second trimester of pregnancy could be much lower than normal. The reduction in hematocrit constitutes the "physiological anemia" of pregnancy. In most cases, investigations as to the true cause of anemia are performed only when the hemoglobin concentration falls below 10/100 ml.

**72. The answer is C.** *(Aladjem, ed 2. pp 7-8.)* Clinical studies have indicated that although systolic blood pressure remains relatively unchanged throughout pregnancy, diastolic blood pressure decreases significantly by the second trimester. A reduction in peripheral vascular resistance, which is noted following the fourteenth week of pregnancy, is responsible for the change in diastolic pressure; this reduction is caused mainly by the increasing percentage of the cardiac output that passes through the uteroplacental circulation.

**73. The answer is E.** *(Aladjem, ed 2. pp 15-17, 23.)* Controlled studies have shown that, during pregnancy, creatinine clearance can vary by ± 50 percent when compared to inulin clearance, the accepted measure of glomerular filtration rate. A higher level of plasma creatinine results in tubular excretion; as a consequence, clearance by the kidney appears to be elevated. Creatinine clearance gives an accurate estimate of glomerular filtration rate only when the latter is less than 20 ml/min.

**74. The answer is B.** *(Aladjem, ed 2. pp 262-266.)* Total urinary estrogens at term are markedly elevated when compared to those of a nonpregnant woman. Estriol constitutes 80 to 85 percent of this urinary estrogen; its precursors are derived from the fetal liver and adrenal glands. When placental sulfatase activity is diminished, urinary excretion of estriol markedly decreases.

**75. The answer is C.** *(Pritchard, ed 16. pp 457-458.)* At the time of delivery, the uterus weighs approximately 1000 g. By 1 week postpartum the weight is down to 500 g; by 4 to 6 weeks postpartum it is back to its normal weight, less than 100 g. Most of the weight loss is due to diminution in cell size rather than cell number. Clinically, it is important to keep these facts in mind when examining patients after delivery. If the uterus is still enlarged at the time of the postpartum checkup (usually at 6 weeks), a pathological process, such as subinvolution of the placental site or retained secundines, should be suspected.

**76. The answer is E.** *(Pritchard, ed 16. pp 465-466.)* Bloody lochia can persist for up to 2 weeks without indicating an underlying pathology; however, if bleeding continues beyond 2 weeks, it may indicate placental site subinvolution, retention of small placental fragments, or both. At this point, appropriate diagnostic and therapeutic measures should be initiated. The physician should first estimate the blood loss and then perform a pelvic examination in search of uterine subinvolution or tenderness. Excessive bleeding or tenderness should lead the physician to suspect retained placental fragments or endometritis. A larger-than-expected but otherwise asymptomatic uterus supports the diagnosis of subinvolution.

Pregnancy, Lactation, and Puerperium    35

77. The answer is D (4). *(Williams, ed 5. p 92.)* Oxytocin causes uterine contractions by an as-yet-unknown mechanism. It does not cause milk production, which is dependent on the presence of insulin, cortisone, estrogen, progesterone, and prolactin; rather, oxytocin stimulates milk ejection by causing myoepithelial cells to contract. Endogenous oxytocin has an extremely mild antidiuretic-hormone effect. When large pharmacological doses of oxytocin are administered, the potential for antidiuresis increases and smooth-muscle relaxation, causing transient hypotension, can occur.

78. The answer is C (2, 4). *(Speroff, ed 2. pp 170-173.)* In the lactating breast, engorgement and milk production begin on the third or fourth postpartum day. Until this time, only colostrum, which is composed of desquamated epithelium and transudate, is manufactured. Transient increases in prolactin levels, which occur after delivery, are initiated by suckling and are crucial to the production of milk; once milk production has begun, however, prolactin levels in lactating as well as nonlactating women return rapidly to low levels. Oxytocin has very little, if any, role in the production of milk. Its primary function in lactation is initiation of milk letdown, which is a neural reflex in which suckling stimulates the myoepithelium of the breast to cause milk to be ejected.

79. The answer is C (2, 4). *(Pritchard, ed 16. pp 236-237, 243, 248.)* Plasma fibrinogen levels increase by about 50 percent during pregnancy. This rise is thought to be at least partially responsible for the great increase in the erythrocyte sedimentation rate. The elevated sedimentation rate is consequently almost useless as a significant laboratory value in pregnant women. Serum albumin decreases by about 30 percent during normal pregnancy. Blood urea nitrogen (BUN) decreases markedly during pregnancy; in fact, BUN values falling in the middle of the normal range for nonpregnant women (i.e., around 10 mg/100 ml) may signal significant impairment of renal function in pregnant women.

80. The answer is E (all). *(Burrow, p 910.)* Methenamine mandelate (Mandelamine), ampicillin, corticosteroids, and phenolphthalein all can reduce urinary estriol levels. Formaldehyde produced by the acid hydrolysis of methenamine mandelate in the urine can degrade estrogens. Hydrolysis of estrogen conjugates is inhibited by phenolphthalein. Large daily doses of cortisol, which can cross the placenta, suppress fetal adrenal function and therefore inhibit production of estriol precursors. Ampicillin use is thought to cause fecal loss of steroids, which results from an inhibition in the gastrointestinal tract of the hydrolysis of biliary estriol conjugates.

81. The answer is C (2, 4). *(Burrow, pp 175-179.)* During pregnancy fasting blood glucose levels generally decrease, probably because the fetus, needing tremendous amounts of glucose, takes glucose at the expense of the mother. In

addition, the maternal response to fasting is accentuated by pregnancy and results in exaggerated starvation ketosis and increased fasting levels of β-hydroxybutyric acid (a ketone body). For a number of reasons, insulin is less effective during pregnancy in diminishing blood glucose. Postprandial blood glucose therefore tends to be higher than in the nonpregnant state, and results of a glucose tolerance test must be interpreted differently. To offset anti-insulin effects, insulin production is augmented during the normal pregnancy, and postprandial insulin levels are increased.

**82. The answer is D (4).** *(Burrow, pp 174-175.)* The tendency for pregnancy to be diabetogenic is thought to be due mainly to the anti-insulin effects of many of the hormones secreted by the placenta as well as to the possible effect of insulin receptors on the placenta itself. Human chorionic somatomammotropin (also known as human placental lactogen) is present in large amounts in the maternal circulation during the third trimester. Its lipolytic and other actions inhibit glucose uptake and manufacture and therefore stimulate insulin production to rise. Levels of pituitary growth hormone are decreased, especially during late pregnancy, and probably have little to do with increased insulin needs. Estrogen and probably progesterone, both of which are present in increased amounts during pregnancy, probably act as peripheral insulin antagonists and therefore would not lead to decreased insulin secretion.

**83. The answer is B (1, 3).** *(Burrow, pp 196-201.)* Probably because of increased estrogen levels, pregnancy is associated with an increase in the amounts of many proteins in the serum, among them thyroxine-binding globulin. In order to maintain normal levels of free thyroxine and triiodothyronine, more total thyroxine must be produced to tie up some of the excess binding sites on the carrier protein. Therefore, the total serum thyroxine concentration increases while the level of free thyroxine stays constant. Thyroid-stimulating hormone (TSH) levels are slightly increased during early pregnancy but by term are back in the normal range, as measured by radioimmunoassay. There are some data to suggest that TSH-like activity also is increased in pregnancy, possibly due to a placental factor, either human chorionic gonadotropin or human chorionic thyrotropin. This explanation applies especially to pregnancies complicated by trophoblastic disease.

**84. The answer is D (4).** *(Yen, pp 159-160.)* Levodopa can cause prolactin secretion to decrease. This compound increases the concentration of dopamine in the hypothalamus and, as a result, probably stimulates production of prolactin-release inhibiting factor. Alpha-methyldopa (which inhibits synthesis of dopamine), phenothiazines, reserpine, and probably serotonin all cause prolactin secretion to increase.

**85. The answer is A (1, 2, 3).** *(Speroff, ed 2. pp 172-173.)* The normal sequence of events triggered by suckling is as follows: through a central-nervous-system response, dopamine is decreased in the hypothalamus. Dopamine suppression decreases production of prolactin inhibitory factor (PIF), which normally travels through a portal system to the pituitary gland; because PIF production is decreased, production of prolactin by the pituitary is increased. At this time, the pituitary also releases oxytocin, which causes milk to be expressed from the alveoli into the lactiferous ducts. Suckling suppresses the production of luteinizing-hormone (LH) releasing factor and, as a result, acts as a mild contraceptive (the midcycle LH surge does not occur).

# PRIMARY CARE

# History, Physical Examination, and Diagnostic Procedures

**DIRECTIONS**: Each question below contains five suggested answers. Choose the **one best** response to each question.

86. The percentage of pregnancy loss that can be attributed to second trimester amniocentesis is

(A) less than 2 percent
(B) 2 to 3 percent
(C) 3 to 4 percent
(D) 5 percent
(E) more than 5 percent

87. A 19-year-old nulliparous woman is given a Venereal Disease Research Laboratories (VDRL) test, which is positive at a dilution of 1:4. The diagnostic measure that now should be ordered is a

(A) Wassermann-type test
(B) rapid plasma reagin card test
(C) fluorescent treponemal antibody-absorption (FTA-ABS) test
(D) lumbar puncture and VDRL titer of cerebrospinal fluid
(E) thorough pelvic examination

88. False positive VDRL tests have been associated with all of the following EXCEPT

(A) narcotic addiction
(B) atypical pneumonias
(C) old age
(D) diabetes mellitus
(E) leprosy

89. All of the following statements concerning a hysterosalpingogram test for fallopian-tube patency are true EXCEPT that

(A) the contrast medium used may be either oil- or water-soluble
(B) salpingitis isthmica nodosa may be diagnosed with this procedure
(C) abnormalities of the uterine cavity may be diagnosed with this procedure
(D) less than 3 ml of contrast medium should be used to avoid spill from the tubes into the peritoneal cavity
(E) the test may have a therapeutic effect on infertility

90. Routine pelvic examination reveals that a 21-year-old woman has a hooded cervix. This finding is most frequently associated with

(A) pregnancy
(B) traumatic abortion
(C) in utero drug exposure
(D) a prior Shirodkar procedure
(E) a herpesvirus infection

91. A woman presents for obstetrical care in the third month of her current pregnancy. Her obstetrical history reveals a spontaneous abortion at 9 weeks gestation, a full-term vaginal delivery, and the delivery of stillborn twins at 24 weeks with each fetus weighing 600 g. She should be classified as a

(A) gravida 3, para 2, abortus 1
(B) gravida 4, para 1, abortus 3
(C) gravida 4, para 2, abortus 1
(D) gravida 4, para 3, abortus 1
(E) gravida 5, para 3, abortus 1

**DIRECTIONS**: Each question below contains four suggested answers of which **one** or **more** is correct. Choose the answer:

| | | | |
|---|---|---|---|
| A | if | 1, 2, and 3 | are correct |
| B | if | 1 and 3 | are correct |
| C | if | 2 and 4 | are correct |
| D | if | 4 | is correct |
| E | if | 1, 2, 3, and 4 | are correct |

92. As a description of a woman's obstetrical history, the digits 7-2-1-6 indicate that she has

(1) given birth to six term infants
(2) had two premature deliveries
(3) been pregnant seven times
(4) had one abortion

93. In recording a gynecological history, 15 x 30 x 6 is a very common way to record the menstrual history. The numbers in this formula include reference to which of the following information?

(1) The woman's age
(2) The interval since the woman's last menstrual period in days
(3) The duration of the woman's last menstrual period in days
(4) The woman's age at her first menses

94. A normal gynecological examination in a 65-year-old woman may yield which of the following findings?

(1) A Bartholin's gland that is nonpalpable
(2) Atrophy of the labia minora
(3) An ovary that is nonpalpable
(4) Dark menstrual-type blood

95. Pelvic examination is an important means of diagnosing ovarian malignancies. An ovarian tumor has an increased likelihood of being malignant if examination reveals that it is

(1) mobile
(2) bilateral
(3) cystic
(4) greater than 10 cm in diameter

96. Injection of labeled dehydroepiandrosterone sulfate into a pregnant woman permits assessment of

(1) fetal adrenal function
(2) placental function
(3) maternal ovarian function
(4) uterine blood flow

97. Routine preoperative evaluation of a patient who has a large, fixed, irregular pelvic mass that is highly suggestive of an ovarian tumor should include which of the following diagnostic procedures?

(1) Chest x-ray
(2) Intravenous pyelography
(3) Barium enema
(4) Liver scan

98. A 23-year-old woman (gravida 2, para 1) wants to know the prenatal diagnosis of her unborn child. Her first child, who was delivered by cesarean section, had anencephaly. An ultrasound examination performed 1 week ago (at 15 weeks gestation) revealed an anterior placenta and a fetal biparietal diameter consistent with the gestational age as determined by menstrual history. In advising the woman, the physician should keep which of the following statements in mind?

(1) An elevated level of alpha-fetoprotein in the amniotic fluid may not necessarily indicate a neural tube defect
(2) An elevated level of alpha-fetoprotein in the amniotic fluid is as likely to indicate a closed neural tube defect as an open neural tube defect
(3) The midtrimester ultrasound examination makes the diagnosis of recurrent anencephaly highly unlikely in this instance
(4) Repeated measurement of the concentration of alpha-fetoprotein in maternal serum can substitute for amniocentesis

99. Analysis of amniotic fluid can be useful in diagnosing which of the following disorders?

(1) Fetal hemolytic anemia
(2) Spina bifida
(3) Postmaturity syndrome
(4) Cleft palate

100. A direct Coombs' test is described by which of the following statements?

(1) It can be useful in analyzing the cord blood of babies at risk for Rh disease
(2) It involves an antiglobulin reagent made by immunizing rabbits to human immunoglobulin
(3) It cannot be used to quantify the amount of an antibody present
(4) It can be performed on the sera of pregnant Rh-negative women to determine the degree of their Rh sensitization

101. A young woman develops painful vulvar vesicles, and a herpesvirus hominis type 2 (herpes simplex) infection is suspected. The tests that can be done to confirm this diagnosis include

(1) wet mount with saline
(2) culture for the virus
(3) Gram stain
(4) Papanicolaou (Pap) smear

Obstetrics and Gynecology

**DIRECTIONS:** The groups of questions below consist of lettered choices followed by several numbered items. For each numbered item select the **one** lettered choice with which it is **most** closely associated. Each lettered choice may be used once, more than once, or not at all.

## Questions 102-104

For each of the descriptions below, select the pelvic type with which it is most likely to be associated.

(A) Anthropoid
(B) Android
(C) Gynecoid
(D) Platypelloid
(E) None of the above

102. Examination of the pelvis reveals prominent ischial spines, a narrow subpubic arch, a narrow high-arched sacrosciatic notch, a straight sacrum, and a shortened posterior sagittal diameter

103. Examination of the pelvis reveals a wide subpubic arch, a curved sacrum, and a shortened anteroposterior diameter

104. Examination of the pelvis reveals a lengthened anteroposterior diameter, a large sacrosciatic notch, prominent ischial spines, and a straight, posteriorly inclined sacrum

## Questions 105-108

For each of the evaluative purposes listed below, select the gynecological procedure that can best be utilized.

(A) Colposcopy
(B) Endometrial biopsy
(C) Laparoscopy
(D) Hysterosalpingography
(E) Culdocentesis

105. Evaluation of patency of the fallopian tubes, the source of pelvic pain, and the occurrence of ovulation

106. Evaluation of abnormal uterine bleeding, the occurrence of ovulation, and abnormal Pap smears

107. Evaluation of patency of the fallopian tubes and intrauterine malformations

108. Evaluation of abnormal uterine bleeding, abnormal Pap smears, and cervical dysplasia

## Questions 109-115

For each condition that follows, select the study that would be helpful in detecting that condition in utero.

(A) Fetal chromosome count
(B) Fetal sex determination
(C) Amniotic fluid level of alpha-fetoprotein
(D) Enzyme analysis of cultured amniotic fluid cells
(E) None of the above

109. Meningomyelocele

110. Achondroplasia

111. Tay-Sachs disease

112. Turner's syndrome

113. Hurler's syndrome

114. Translocation Down's syndrome

115. Hydrocephaly (without associated spinal cord defects)

# History, Physical Examination, and Diagnostic Procedures Answers

**86. The answer is A.** *(The NICHD National Registry for Amniocentesis Study Group, JAMA 236:1471-1476, 1976. Working Party of Amniocentesis, Br J Obstet Gynaecol 85:2, 1978.)* A national prospective controlled study, designed to evaluate the safety and accuracy of prenatal genetic diagnosis by early midtrimester amniocentesis, revealed that the incidence of fetal loss in the approximately 1000 women studied did not differ significantly from that of the controls. The incidence of pregnancy loss directly attributable to midtrimester amniocentesis was found to be less than 1 percent. This finding has been confirmed by a similar study conducted in Canada. The overall accuracy of midtrimester amniocentesis for prenatal genetic diagnosis was found to be 99.4 percent. A British study, however, found a higher 2.6 percent rate of fetal loss with amniocentesis as compared with a 1.1 percent rate in the control group.

**87. The answer is C.** *(Monif, pp 176-177.)* Because a positive VDRL test either may indicate the presence of syphilis or may be a biological false positive, a specific treponemal test, such as the fluorescent treponemal antibody-absorption (FTA-ABS) test, is needed to discriminate false positives from true infection. The rapid plasma reagin (RPR) card test and Wassermann-type tests, such as the Kolmer test, are nontreponemal tests and therefore are no more specific than the VDRL test. A lumbar puncture would not be indicated at this point. A pelvic examination may be of little diagnostic use, because chancres often disappear before a VDRL test becomes positive.

**88. The answer is D.** *(Parsons, ed 2. p 869.)* The VDRL is a serological test widely used to screen for syphilis. False positives appear in approximately 3 to 4 percent of all VDRL tests performed. If a false positive occurs, a physician first should ensure that the result is not due to technical error and second should consider the various entities that result in false positives at the following rates:

History, Physical, and Diagnosis    47

leprosy (8 to 28 percent), smallpox vaccination (1 to 2 pereent), narcotic addiction (20 to 25 percent), and old age (10 percent of patients between 70 and 80 years of age). Atypical pneumonias have also resulted in false positives. The FTA-ABS treponemal test, which is quite specific, should be used with a borderline or suspected false positive VDRL test.

**89. The answer is D.** *(Speroff, ed 2. pp 323-324.)* A hysterosalpingogram is a procedure in which 3 to 6 ml of either an oil- or water-soluble contrast medium is injected through the cervix in order to outline the uterine cavity and fallopian tubes. Spill of contrast medium into the peritoneal cavity proves patency of the uterine cavity and fallopian tubes. By outlining the cavity, abnormalities such as bicornuate uterus, uterine polyps, submucous myomas, salpingitis isthmica nodosum, and hydrosalpinx can be identified. Some controlled studies have shown a therapeutic effect resulting in an increased rate of pregnancy in infertility patients.

**90. The answer is C.** *(Herbst, Clin Obstet Gynecol 18:185-194, 1975.)* A hooded cervix, a "cockscomb" cervix, and cervical pseudopolyps are common structural changes associated with in utero exposure to diethylstilbestrol or chemically related nonsteroidal estrogens. Cervical erosions are almost always found in affected individuals, and vaginal adenosis is frequently present. Carcinomas of the vagina are much less frequently diagnosed.

**91. The answer is C.** *(Wynn, ed 2. pp 4-5.)* Gravidity refers to the total number of times a woman has been pregnant, regardless of the outcome, and includes the present pregnancy. Parity refers to the number of births, alive or dead, that weigh 500 g or more. When the weight is unknown, an estimated gestational age of 20 weeks or more is used to define parity. Multiple gestations are counted as one birth. Spontaneous or induced termination of a pregnancy prior to 20 weeks of gestation is recorded as an abortus.

**92. The answer is C (2, 4).** *(Pritchard, ed 16. p 304.)* Describing an obstetrical history by the four-digit system is more comprehensive than merely indicating gravidity and parity. The first digit of the four indicates the number of term infants delivered; the second, the number of premature infants delivered; the third, the number of abortions; and the fourth, the number of children now alive. A woman described as 7-2-1-6, therefore, has had seven term deliveries, two premature deliveries, and one abortion; and six of her children currently are alive.

93. **The answer is D (4).** *(Wynn, ed 2. pp 5-6.)* The formula 15 x 30 x 6 is a commonly used abbreviation for recording a woman's menstrual history. The first digit refers to the woman's age at the onset of menses (menarche). The second digit refers to the usual interval between menses in days. The third digit refers to the duration of the woman's usual menstrual period in days. Thus, the woman described by this formula was 15 years of age at the onset of menses; her cycle runs approximately 30 days; and each period lasts approximately 6 days.

94. **The answer is A (1, 2, 3).** *(Wynn, ed 2. pp 15-19.)* The Bartholin's gland located at the junction of the middle and lower thirds of the vagina is usually not palpable unless it is involved in a cyst or an abscess. The decreased estrogen levels associated with the postmenopausal state are normally associated with atrophic changes of the labia minora, vaginal mucosa, uterus, and ovaries. It is common to be unable to palpate the normal ovary, especially in an obese, uncooperative, or postmenopausal woman. Any bleeding whatsoever in the postmenopausal female should be considered abnormal and should alert the physician to the possibility of a malignancy.

95. **The answer is C (2, 4).** *(DiSaia, p 141.)* Unilateral, cystic, mobile, and small (less than 10 cm) adnexal masses tend to be benign neoplasms. Masses that are bilateral, solid, fixed, and large, on the other hand, more characteristically are malignant and require prompt diagnostic evaluation and treatment. Ascites also is frequently associated with ovarian malignancies.

96. **The answer is C (2, 4).** *(Burrow, p 912.)* Less than 0.2 percent of circulating dehydroepiandrosterone sulfate (DS) is converted to estrogen by nonpregnant women. In late pregnancy, however, the placenta converts from 75 to 80 percent of maternal circulating DS to estrone and estradiol. The clearance rate of labeled DS is felt to reflect uterine blood flow, and the production of labeled estradiol is an indicator of placental function.

97. **The answer is A (1, 2, 3).** *(DiSaia, pp 142-145.)* A chest x-ray, an intravenous pyelogram, and a barium enema all are important in the evaluation of a woman suspected of having an ovarian malignancy. Chest x-rays can reveal occult metastases as well as pleural effusions, which frequently occur in advanced ovarian cancer. Pyelography can assess renal function and reveal ureteral obstruction or deviation as well as duplication of urinary-tract structures. Barium enemas can help distinguish a neoplastic or inflammatory process arising from the colon from extrinsic compression due to an ovarian tumor. A liver scan is not routinely performed, because ovarian cancer usually does not spread hematogenously; a scan is indicated only if liver function tests are abnormal or the liver is palpably enlarged.

History, Physical, and Diagnosis                                    49

**98. The answer is B (1, 3).** *(Pritchard, ed 16. pp 339-344.)* The demonstration by ultrasound examination of a well-defined vertex of normal size can rule out anencephaly. Amniotic fluid levels of alpha-fetoprotein are currently the most reliable tool to detect those neural tube defects not covered by skin (open defects). Elevated levels also may be associated with fetal blood contamination of the amniotic fluid (often due to amniocentesis through an anteriorly implanted placenta) or with a number of fetal disorders. Because maternal serum alpha-fetoprotein levels have been reported to be elevated in only 50 to 70 percent of cases in which the fetus has had an open neural tube defect, its use as the exclusive diagnostic procedure in couples at increased risk for having children with this disorder is not generally recommended.

**99. The answer is A (1, 2, 3).** *(Burrow, pp 918-923.)* Because spectrophotometric analysis of amniotic fluid can determine the concentration of indirect bilirubin, which is a reflection of fetal red cell hemolysis, the procedure is a mainstay in the management of patients who have Rh incompatibility. If meconium is present in amniotic fluid aspirated from a pregnant woman who is at least 2 weeks past her due date, the presence of postmaturity syndrome must be assumed until proven otherwise. Open neural tube defects, such as spina bifida, can be diagnosed by the high levels of alpha-fetoprotein in the amniotic fluid; closed neural tube defects, on the other hand, are not accompanied by increased concentrations of this substance. Cleft palate cannot be diagnosed at this time by chromosomal or biochemical analyses of amniotic fluid.

**100. The answer is A (1, 2, 3).** *(Queenan, ed 2. pp 14-15.)* The direct Coombs' test, which uses human antiglobulin derived from immunized rabbits, is performed on blood cells to determine if they are coated with antibody. A direct Coombs' test, therefore, can be useful in analyzing the cord blood of an infant who is at risk for Rh disease. Quantification of antibody titers can be achieved by doing serial dilutions of the indirect Coombs' test, which analyzes serum.

**101. The answer is C (2, 4).** *(Monif, pp 56-57.)* Herpesvirus hominis type 2 (herpes simplex) can be cultured readily and rapidly; however, available facilities to perform viral cultures are limited. A Papanicolaou (Pap) smear will show typical herpetic findings (multinucleated giant cells and intranuclear inclusions) in approximately 85 percent of affected women. Wet mounts and Gram stains are inadequate detectors of viral infection.

**102-104. The answers are: 102-B, 103-D, 104-A.** *(Pritchard, ed 16. pp 286-288.)* The four general pelvic configurations, named here according to the widely used Caldwell-Moloy classification, may be important indicators of potential problems during labor and delivery. The gynecoid pelvis, the most common type, is generally round, with the transverse diameter being the same as or slightly greater than the anteroposterior diameter.

The anthropoid pelvis is essentially oblong, with the anteroposterior diameter being much greater than the transverse diameter. It is thus a deep, narrow pelvis; characteristically, the ischial spines are prominent and the sacrum is inclined posteriorly.

The android pelvis is often described as triangular. The anterior pelvis is narrowed, with a narrow subpubic angle; but, unlike the anthropoid pelvis, the posterior pelvis is short, with a small posterior sagittal diameter. The spines are prominent in the android pelvis, and the sacrum is straight. Unless it is unusually large, this type of pelvis offers a poor prognosis for delivery.

The rarest pelvic type is the platypelloid ("flat") pelvis. Here the anteroposterior diameter is quite short and the transverse diameter is wide. The subpubic angle is wide and the ischial spines are not prominent. This type of pelvis may cause the vertex to stay in the occiput transverse position until delivery.

**105-108. The answers are: 105-C, 106-B, 107-D, 108-A.** *(Wynn, ed 2. pp 129-132.)* **Colposcopy** is an office procedure for examination of the cervix at 10 to 40 x magnification. The technique can reveal cervical abnormalities, including neoplasia in its intraepithelial stages. Colposcopy is therefore useful in evaluating patients with abnormal Pap smears and abnormal uterine bleeding. An **endometrial biopsy** is an office procedure that is helpful in identifying the occurrence of ovulation by observing a progestational effect on the endometrium. It is also used in evaluating patients with an abnormal Pap smear or abnormal bleeding for the presence of endometrial neoplasia. **Laparoscopy** is an operating room procedure in which a telescopic instrument is inserted through the abdominal wall after the peritoneal cavity is distended with gas. It has many diagnostic purposes, such as evaluation of infertility, tubal patency, the occurrence of ovulation, pelvic pain, pelvic masses, and suspected cases of intra-abdominal hemorrhage. Laparoscopy is also utilized for therapeutic purposes, such as lysis of adhesions, cauterization of endometriosis, and tubal ligation. **Hysterosalpingography** involves the injection of a radiopaque fluid through the cervical canal; the uterine and tubal cavities are thus outlined for visualization radiologically. With hysterosalpingography infertile patients can be evaluated for tubal patency and uterine malformations. **Culdocentesis** is an office procedure in which a needle is inserted through the posterior vaginal wall in an attempt to sample intraperitoneal fluid from Douglas' cul-de-sac. It is therefore useful in identifying the presence or absence of intraperitoneal blood, pus, and exfoliating neoplastic cells.

History, Physical, and Diagnosis 51

**109-115. The answers are: 109-C, 110-E, 111-D, 112-A, 113-D, 114-E, 115-E.** *(Burrow, p 810. Golbus, Obstet Gynecol 48:497, 1976.)* Aneuploidy can be detected simply by counting fetal chromosomes; the diagnosis of aneuploid disorders, such as Turner's syndrome (45,XO) and trisomy 21 (classic Down's syndrome) can be confirmed by karyotype. Because individuals who have translocation Down's syndrome have 46 chromosomes, a chromosome count would be unrewarding; modern chromosome-banding techniques, however, can demonstrate this abnormality during analysis of the karyotype. Although achondroplasia is an inherited, autosomal dominant disorder, it cannot be detected by karyotypic analysis at this time.

Meningomyelocele and other open neural-tube defects have markedly elevated amniotic fluid levels of alpha-fetoprotein, probably as a result of the transudation of this protein across the membrane covering the defect. If a neural-tube defect is completely covered with skin, however, the alpha-fetoprotein level may be within normal limits; an example of such closed defects is hydrocephaly that is not associated with spinal cord lesions.

Tay-Sachs disease results from a defect in the synthesis of hexosaminidase A. Hurler's syndrome is caused by a deficiency of the enzyme α-L-iduronidase. Both disorders can be detected by enzyme analysis of cultured fetal cells grown from amniotic fluid.

# Clinical, Behavioral, Medical, and Legal Problems

**DIRECTIONS**: Each question below contains five suggested answers. Choose the one **best** response to each question.

116. Labial agglutination in a young girl is best treated by

(A) forcible separation
(B) estrogen cream
(C) surgical excision
(D) antibiotics
(E) warm compresses

117. The most common cause of precocious puberty in girls is

(A) idiopathic
(B) gonadal tumors
(C) Albright's syndrome
(D) hypothyroidism
(E) central nervous system tumors

118. Which of the following statements about congenital adrenal hyperplasia is true?

(A) It is most commonly seen and recognized in newborn males
(B) The genetic defect is an autosomal recessive gene
(C) The most common form of the syndrome is due to 11-$\beta$-hydroxylase deficiency
(D) Salt wasting and hypertension are present in all cases
(E) Heterozygous carriers can easily be detected

119. Which of the following statements is true regarding the menarchial female?

(A) Pubic hair growth generally precedes breast budding
(B) Most cycles are anovulatory in the first year of menstruation
(C) Body weight correlates highly with the onset of menarche
(D) The age of menarche bears little association with mother's age of menarche
(E) The mean age of menarche in this country is increasing slightly with each decade

120. Which of the following statements about precocious puberty in girls is true?

(A) It signifies ovulatory capability
(B) It often is heralded by a growth spurt
(C) Menarche is usually the first symptom
(D) Fertility tests are crucial for affected girls
(E) True sexual precocity cannot stem from neoplastic causes

121. The management of girls who have idiopathic precocious puberty includes

(A) progestin therapy
(B) estrogen therapy
(C) androgen therapy
(D) pelvic irradiation
(E) laparoscopy

122. A 17-year-old girl presents at the emergency room at 6 A.M. with acute urinary retention. On questioning, she states that her menstrual periods have not started, although she does have a monthly attack of mild lower abdominal discomfort, which is relieved by analgesics. Physical examination reveals well-developed secondary sexual characteristics, with an abdominal mass extending up to the level of the umbilicus. A pregnancy test is negative. The most likely diagnosis is

(A) intrauterine fetal death
(B) imperforate hymen
(C) ovarian tumor
(D) tuberculous peritonitis
(E) gestational trophoblastic disease

123. The most frequent cause of a bloody discharge from the nipple is

(A) carcinoma of the breast
(B) intraductal papilloma
(C) fibroadenoma
(D) cystosarcoma phyllodes
(E) breast abscess

124. In the experience of Masters and Johnson and other sex therapists, the sexual dysfunction having the lowest cure rate is

(A) premature ejaculation
(B) vaginismus
(C) primary impotence
(D) secondary impotence
(E) female orgasmic dysfunction

125. A 46-year-old woman presents with depression, urinary urgency, night sweats, and headaches. On examination she is found to be anovulatory. The most likely diagnosis is

(A) psychosomatic disorder
(B) manic depression
(C) urinary tract infection
(D) tuberculosis with renal involvement
(E) menopause

126. A 22-year-old woman, gravida 3, para 2 (one abortion), is brought to the hospital because she says she has been raped by a 35-year-old man whom she knows to have had a vasectomy 2 years ago. Both individuals have an A-positive blood type. Which of the following would be most useful to her in the prosecution of this case?

(A) Accurate description of the introitus
(B) Smear for sperm from the cervix
(C) Vaginal washings for acid phosphatase
(D) Specific typing of vaginal washings
(E) Examination of her pubic hair

**DIRECTIONS**: Each question below contains four suggested answers of which **one** or **more** is correct. Choose the answer:

| A | if | 1, 2, and 3 | are correct |
|---|---|---|---|
| B | if | 1 and 3 | are correct |
| C | if | 2 and 4 | are correct |
| D | if | 4 | is correct |
| E | if | 1, 2, 3, and 4 | are correct |

127. The following chromosomal complements are all associated with gonadal dysgenesis. Short stature is characteristic in

(1) XO
(2) XXp-
(3) XXqi
(4) XXq-

128. Risk factors for the development of breast cancer include

(1) breast cancer in premenopausal first-degree relatives
(2) breast cancer in postmenopausal first-degree relatives
(3) previous mastectomy
(4) childbearing

129. True statements regarding the diagnosis of breast disease include which of the following?

(1) Breast examination is an integral part of the gynecological examination
(2) Ambulatory facilities for breast biopsy are not cost effective
(3) Women should be taught how and when to examine their own breasts
(4) Surgical referral is preferable to initiating diagnostic procedures

130. Endocrine-related causes of short stature in young women include

(1) hypothyroidism
(2) adrenal hyperplasia
(3) Cushing's disease
(4) Turner's syndrome

131. The use of estrogen replacement therapy may be hazardous, if not expressly contraindicated, for women who have

(1) impaired hepatic function
(2) thromboembolic disorders
(3) estrogen-dependent tumors
(4) a mother or sister with osteoporosis

132. Side effects of estrogen replacement therapy include which of the following?

(1) Vaginitis
(2) Edema
(3) Weight loss
(4) Breast tenderness

133. Estrogen administration is considered advantageous in the treatment of perimenopausal women who have

(1) emotional reactions
(2) vasomotor reactions
(3) osteoporosis
(4) epithelial atrophy

134. True statements regarding breast cancer include which of the following?

(1) Carcinoma of the breast is the most common malignancy in women in the Western world
(2) Cancer of the breast and genital organs accounts for nearly 75 percent of all new cancers in women
(3) Approximately 90,000 new cases of breast cancer are diagnosed in the United States each year
(4) One woman in six will develop breast cancer

135. Psychological manifestations of the menopause include

(1) emotional lability
(2) insomnia
(3) irritability
(4) fatigue

136. Female dyspareunia can be described by which of the following statements?

(1) It rarely affects postmenopausal women
(2) Complaints of pain during penile thrusting usually indicate pelvic pathology
(3) Bacterial vaginal infection is a minor etiological factor
(4) It can develop from sensitivity to intravaginal contraceptive agents

137. Diabetes, because it is a systemic disease that can affect vascular and neurological function, often alters sexual performance. Problems commonly encountered by diabetic individuals include

(1) frequent vaginal infections in women
(2) simultaneous onset of impotence and decrease of libido in men
(3) loss of previously established orgasmic capacity in women
(4) loss of vaginal contractions during orgasm in women

138. Primary orgasmic dysfunction in women can be described by which of the following statements?

(1) It can stem from dissatisfaction with a partner's behavior patterns
(2) The influence of orthodox religious beliefs is still of major etiological significance
(3) It can be exacerbated if a partner suffers from premature ejaculation
(4) A woman affected by it has never in her life achieved orgasm

139. The syndrome of vaginismus is described by which of the following statements?

(1) It involves involuntary reflex contraction of the vaginal musculature
(2) It is rarely associated with concomitant dysfunction in the male partner
(3) Affected women can be helped by the use of vaginal dilators
(4) Diagnosis can be definitely established by history

| SUMMARY OF DIRECTIONS | | | | |
|---|---|---|---|---|
| A | B | C | D | E |
| 1, 2, 3 only | 1, 3 only | 2, 4 only | 4 only | All are correct |

140. A man and a woman, both 70 years old, consult a sex therapist because of the man's impotence. The woman first became concerned when he failed to ejaculate on several occasions and the man finally agreed that therapy was needed when his erections disappeared completely (except for occasional erections upon awakening). The therapist should tell the couple that

(1) the man's morning erections are not an indication that his physiological sexual response is intact
(2) older men frequently experience orgasm without ejaculation
(3) the loss of the ability to have an erection is a normal consequence of the aging process
(4) ejaculatory demand decreases with age

141. Masters and Johnson interviewed 331 women concerning their attitudes toward sexual activity during menstruation. This study revealed that

(1) approximately 20 percent of these women objected to it on aesthetic grounds
(2) approximately 50 percent of these women were positively interested in it
(3) approximately 20 percent of these women objected to it on religious grounds
(4) many women's attitudes were affected by the opinions of their male partners

142. Although the incidence of rape is increasing in the United States, data indicate that three out of every four rapes still are not reported to law enforcement authorities. True statements about rape include which of the following?

(1) Rape usually results in pregnancy
(2) Many rapes are perpetrated by men who find violence necessary for sexual fulfillment
(3) Tests for venereal disease should not be performed on rape victims immediately following a rape
(4) Rape can cause sexual dysfunction

# Behavioral, Medical, and Legal Problems

**DIRECTIONS**: The group of questions below consists of lettered choices followed by several numbered items. For each numbered item select the **one** lettered choice with which it is **most** closely associated. Each lettered choice may be used once, more than once, or not at all.

## Questions 143-147

For each of the circumstances of death that might occur in a patient with generalized carcinomatosis, select the correct term used to describe the occurrence.

(A) Natural death
(B) Passive euthanasia
(C) Active euthanasia
(D) Facilitated suicide
(E) Suicide

143. Coincidental myocardial infarction with failure of resuscitative efforts

144. Overdose of barbiturates procured by the patient and administered by the patient without the physician's consent

145. Overdose of barbiturates procured by the physician and administered by the patient with the physician's and patient's consent

146. Overdose of barbiturates procured by the physician and administered by the physician with the physician's and patient's consent

147. Myocardial infarction with no attempt at resuscitative efforts

# Clinical, Behavioral, Medical, and Legal Problems

## Answers

**116. The answer is B.** *(Green, ed 3. p 121.)* Labial agglutination is a condition in young girls in which the labia minora are fused together. There is no relationship to either hygiene or presence of vulvovaginitis, and generally speaking the exact reason for the agglutination is unknown. It is important, however, to distinguish this condition from possible congenital anomalies. In asymptomatic patients, no treatment is necessary other than reassurance as this condition will resolve with estrogen production at puberty; however, in patients with symptoms, such as local irritation or difficulty in micturition, separation can be achieved with constant application of estrogen creams. Surgical or forcible separation of the labia should be avoided. Antibiotics and warm compresses are ineffective.

**117. The answer is A.** *(Speroff, ed 2. pp 255-258.)* In North America, any pubertal changes before the age of 8 years in girls and 9 years in boys are regarded as precocious. Although the most common type of precocious puberty in girls is idiopathic, it is essential to ensure close long-term follow-up of these patients to ascertain that there is no serious underlying pathology, such as tumors of the central nervous system or ovary. Only 1 to 2 percent of patients with precocious puberty have an estrogen-producing ovarian tumor as the causative factor. Albright's syndrome (polyostotic fibrous dysplasia) is also relatively rare and consists of fibrous dysplasia and cystic degeneration of the long bones, sexual precocity, and café au lait spots on the skin. Hypothyroidism is a cause of precocious puberty in some children, making thyroid function tests mandatory in these cases. Central nervous system tumors as a cause of precocious puberty occur more commonly in boys than in girls.

**118. The answer is B.** *(Speroff, ed 2. pp 236-240.)* Congenital adrenal hyperplasia accounts for 40 to 50 percent of all infants with ambiguous genitalia. It is most commonly seen and recognized in newborn females. At birth, the characteristic abnormalities of the genitalia include clitoral enlargement and various degrees of vulvar fusion in the female; in the male, hypospadias and bilateral cryptorchidism are common features. There is a strong familial tendency, with the

Behavioral, Medical, and Legal Problems 59

genetic defect being an autosomal recessive gene. 21-Hydroxylase deficiency is the most common form of congenital adrenal hyperplasia, with 11-β-hydroxylase deficiency associated with the hypertensive form. The salt-wasting variety is related to the degree of enzyme block in the 21-hydroxylase deficiency type. Fatal cases are associated with the 3-β-dehydrogenase and 20-, 22-hydroxylase deficiencies.

**119. The answer is C.** *(Romney, ed 2. pp 385-386.)* Although the exact mechanism of menarche is not clearly understood, there is strong evidence to suggest that body weight is the critical variable. There is a high degree of correlation with the growth pattern and the age of menarche of the mother and other female relatives. Menarche occurs approximately 1 to 1 1/2 years after the onset of pubic hair and about 2 years after the appearance of breast buds. Although menses are frequently irregular in the first year or two, studies show that approximately half of the cycles are ovulatory.

**120. The answer is B.** *(Speroff, ed 2. pp 255-256.)* Precocious puberty is usually heralded by an earlier-than-expected growth spurt. Although it most commonly is idiopathic or constitutional, sexual precocity, even if accompanied by ovulation and progesterone production, can be brought on by certain disease states, such as tumors of the ovary or central nervous system. Menarche may appear as the initial symptom of precocious puberty; more often, however, it is a late symptom, depending on the production of high levels of gonadotropins over a period of time. Ovulatory capability does not necessarily accompany sexual development, and tests for fertility, such as progesterone assays, usually are not necessary.

**121. The answer is A.** *(Speroff, ed 2. p 259.)* Progestin therapy is the treatment of choice for girls who have idiopathic precocious puberty. Although progestins cannot cause pubic hair to disappear, they can stop future growth, arrest breast development, and, most important, cause bone growth to decelerate, thus preventing early epiphyseal closure. Progestin treatment should be stopped when bone age equals chronological age. Estrogen therapy is contraindicated because it can only exacerbate symptoms of precocity and result in short stature. Laparoscopy is not indicated, because most causes of precocious puberty can eventually be determined without surgery.

**122. The answer is B.** *(Jeffcoate, ed 4. p 142.)* Patients with imperforate hymen may present to the physician seeking an explanation for amenorrhea; however, in many instances such patients may present as an emergency with abdominal pain with or without an abdominopelvic mass. The intact hymen results in the retention of menstrual blood, which may accumulate over time (often 3 to 4 years). This accumulation of blood in the vagina, uterus, and tubes may result in a pelvic mass that may in turn cause a mechanical obstruction of the urethra. Thus, acute urinary retention with a distended bladder may be the patient's presenting symptoms.

123. **The answer is B.** *(Green, ed 3. pp 616-618.)* Fibroadenomas are the most common benign breast tumors, and they usually do not give rise to any significant symptoms. The diagnosis is often made by the physician on routine examination of the breasts. Intraductal papilloma is the second most common benign breast tumor. Its presenting sign is that of a bloody discharge from the nipple. In order to rule out possible underlying intraductal papillary adenocarcinoma, intraductal papilloma is often treated surgically. Cystosarcoma phyllodes is also a benign tumor that rarely undergoes malignant changes. It can grow to a very large size and surgery is again the recommended treatment. Cancer of the breast can also give rise to a bloody nipple discharge, although not as commonly as intraductal papilloma. A breast abscess may give rise to a purulent nipple discharge.

124. **The answer is C.** *(Masters, 1970. p 367.)* In a 5-year follow-up study of couples treated by Masters and Johnson, the cure rates for vaginismus and premature ejaculation approached 100 percent. Orgasmic dysfunction was corrected in 80 percent of women, and secondary impotence (impotence despite a history of previous coital success) resolved in 70 percent of men. Primary impotence (chronic and complete inability to maintain an erection sufficient for coitus) was cured only 60 percent of the time. Other therapists report very similar statistics.

125. **The answer is E.** *(Speroff, ed 2. pp 77-78.)* The symptoms described in the question are common symptoms of menopause. They all result primarily from estrogen withdrawal, and most can be reversed by estrogen therapy. "Climacteric" is actually a better word for this complex of symptoms, because the menopause is technically the instant at which menses cease.

126. **The answer is C.** *(American College of Obstetricians and Gynecologists, ACOG Tech Bull 14: July, 1972.)* Although all of the procedures mentioned in the question can be helpful in establishing a case of rape in most situations, the expected lack of sperm and the matching blood types in the situation presented would limit their value in this case. Only the finding of 50 units/ml or more of acid phosphatase in this woman's vagina could be taken as evidence of ejaculation. Her introitus probably would not be injured because of her parity. Foreign pubic hair might only indicate close contact.

Behavioral, Medical, and Legal Problems 61

**127. The answer is A (1, 2, 3).** *(Speroff, ed 2. p 245.)* It is believed that the genes controlling both stature and the other stigmata of Turner's syndrome are located on the short arm of the X chromosome. Accordingly, XO or a deletion of the X short arm (XXp-) or a long arm X isochromosome (XXqi), where the entire short arm of X is deleted, will give rise to short stature. The deletion of the X long arm (XXq-) gives rise to patients with streak gonads but normal stature.

**128. The answer is A (1, 2, 3).** *(Ryan, p 364.)* First-degree relatives (mothers, sisters, and daughters) of a premenopausal woman with unilateral breast cancer have a 3 times increased risk of developing breast cancer, while the same tumor discovered after menopause gives a 1.5 times increased risk to first-degree relatives. In a woman with a previous mastectomy the likelihood of a second primary in the remaining breast is approximately 10 to 15 percent and increases at a rate of 1 percent per year. Childbearing, especially prior to 30 years of age, decreases the risk of breast cancer in the female.

**129. The answer is B (1, 3).** *(Ryan, p 362.)* The American College of Obstetricians and Gynecologists released a policy statement in 1978 which confirmed the pivotal role played by the specialist in reproductive medicine in the early detection and diagnosis of breast disease. This role includes the initiation of specific diagnostic procedures such as needle aspiration and mammography. In this regard, the use of ambulatory facilities for diagnostic workup is both appropriate and cost effective. Examination of the breasts is an essential part of the gynecological examination, and in addition the patient should be instructed in the technique of self-examination for those times between visits to her physician.

**130. The answer is E (all).** *(Speroff, ed 2. pp 260-261.)* Short stature can be associated with adrenal hyperplasia, Cushing's disease, and exogenous cortisone therapy. These factors cause short stature by increasing cortisol levels and, as a result, stimulating epiphyseal closure. Individuals who have Turner's syndrome also are characterized by short stature, due to a lack of estrogen production. Hypothyroidism and hypopituitarism can cause short stature in affected girls.

**131. The answer is A (1, 2, 3).** *(Speroff, ed 2. pp 83-85.)* The use of estrogen replacement therapy can be deleterious for women who have thromboembolic symptoms. Because the liver is influenced significantly by estrogens, which can affect the function of hepatic cell enzymes and production of lipids and lipoproteins, the effects of hepatic impairment can be exacerbated by estrogen therapy. The existence of estrogen-dependent tumors is a contraindication to estrogen use. The long-term disabilities of osteoporosis may be ameliorated with estrogen therapy.

**132. The answer is C (2, 4).** *(Speroff, ed 2. p 85.)* Side effects of estrogen replacement therapy can include edema, weight gain, increased vaginal bleeding, and breast tenderness. Development of these side effects usually occurs in conjunction with inappropriately high doses of estrogen. Vaginitis, along with dyspareunia, dysuria, pruritus, and other symptoms, is associated with decreased levels of estrogen.

**133. The answer is E (all).** *(Speroff, ed 2. pp 80-83.)* There is good evidence that estrogen reduces anxiety, depression, and other emotional reactions that can accompany menopause. Estrogens also are helpful in retarding osteoporosis, although their use cannot replace the calcium that already has been lost. The clearest response to estrogen therapy is by the autonomic nervous system; relief from vasomotor reactions, such as hot flashes, by the use of estrogens is significant. A variety of other disturbing symptoms related to epithelial atrophy, such as dyspareunia and urinary urgency, may also be reversed with estrogen therapy.

**134. The answer is B (1, 3).** *(Ryan, pp 363-364.)* In females of the Western world, carcinoma of the breast has become, by far, the most common form of malignancy. Data from the National Cancer Institute reveal an incidence of 70 to 76 per 100,000 white American females. The reported incidence is slightly lower, 60 to 61 per 100,000, in black American females. This means that 1 in every 13 females will develop breast cancer at some time in her life. Breast cancers and cancers of the female genital tract together account for approximately 50 percent of all new cancers reported each year. Because of this relatively high frequency, screening programs for early detection, such as self-examination of breasts and Papanicolaou (Pap) smears, can have a significant impact on the overall outcome of this disease.

**135. The answer is E (all).** *(Ryan, p 437.)* Menopausal women may express emotional lability under stress as irritability, depression, or anxiety. A manifestation of the depression is insomnia with fatigue. It remains to be clarified how much of the psychological manifestations of the menopause is related to the central effects of estrogen deprivation and how much is due to the "empty nest" syndrome and the woman's sociologically influenced expectations of the menopause.

**136. The answer is D (4).** *(Masters, 1970. pp 266-288.)* Aside from psychological causes, female dyspareunia also can stem from a number of physical disorders. Infection of the vaginal barrel, such as with *Escherichia coli* or *Streptococcus faecalis*, can cause distressing burning and aching during and after coition. Insufficient vaginal lubrication also can cause dyspareunia; this condition can occur in postmenopausal women who are not receiving estrogen replacement therapy. Sensitivity to intravaginal chemical contraceptives and irritation of the clitoris, vaginal outlet, or labia can lead to dyspareunia. A woman's complaint of pain during penile thrusting is difficult to evaluate; although this pain can indicate pelvic disorders, such as laceration of uterine ligaments, it also frequently stems from a desire to avoid intercourse.

**137. The answer is B (1, 3).** *(Ellenberg, Ann Intern Med 75:213-219, 1971. Kolodny, Diabetes 20:557-559, 1971. Lief, pp 117-118.)* The susceptibility of diabetic women to fungal and bacterial vaginitis, which can cause irritation during coitus, may be a contributing factor in the disappearance of the orgasmic response that occurs in about 30 percent of women who have diabetes. Neurological factors, however, have not been adequately explored. There is no evidence that orgasm, when it does occur, differs between diabetic and nondiabetic women. Men who have diabetes may notice diminished erectile capacity as much as a year before diabetes becomes clinically evident; libido generally remains unimpaired.

**138. The answer is E (all).** *(Masters, 1970. pp 227-237.)* Many factors can contribute to the development of primary orgasmic dysfunction in women. By definition, these women will not have been able to achieve orgasm through any physical means at any time in their lives; reasons for their dysfunction can include the influence of orthodox religious beliefs, dissatisfaction with their partners' behavioral or social traits, past trauma (such as rape), or rigid familial sexual proscriptions. Sexual dysfunction, particularly premature ejaculation, in a male partner can reinforce a woman's orgasmic dysfunction.

**139. The answer is B (1, 3).** *(Masters, 1970. pp 250-251, 262-265.)* Vaginismus is defined as the involuntary spastic contraction of the muscles surrounding the vaginal orifice. Although a history of vaginal "tightness" and pain on entry is highly suggestive of the condition, the diagnosis must be verified by demonstrating involuntary spasm on pelvic examination. A large proportion of the partners of affected women have primary or secondary impotence. Counseling and the use of vaginal dilators can be highly successful in treating women who have vaginismus.

**140. The answer is D (4).** *(Masters, 1970. pp 322-325.)* The presence of morning erections indicates adequate physiological sexual capacity and remains the best historical guide for screening men complaining of impotence. The capacity for erection generally persists into old age, unless directly interfered with by medications or medical illness. More lengthy and direct genital stimulation may be needed for an older man to attain full erection. The feeling of a need to ejaculate ("ejaculatory demand") decreases with age. If one or both sexual partners feel that coitus is incomplete without ejaculation, feelings of inadequacy can develop, leading ultimately to impotence. Orgasm is almost invariably accompanied by ejaculation.

**141. The answer is C (2, 4).** *(Masters, 1966. pp 125-126.)* Masters and Johnson interviewed 331 women concerning their attitudes toward sexual activity during menstruation. Of these women, approximately 10 percent objected to sexual activity at this time based on religious and aesthetic considerations. Approximately 50 percent of the women were positively interested in sexual activity, especially during the latter half of menstruation, and the remaining women were essentially indifferent provided that they felt well, were not menstruating heavily, and felt there were no aesthetic objections from their male partners. Approximately 13 percent of the women felt that sexual activity decreased dysmenorrhea, and Masters and Johnson clinically demonstrated that sexual activity during menstruation in fact caused a uterine contractile response and temporarily increased the rate of menstrual flow.

**142. The answer is C (2, 4).** *(American Medical Association Committee on Human Sexuality, pp 138-139.)* Although rape does not usually cause pregnancy, it can result in numerous emotional and physical sequelae, including sexual dysfunction, venereal disease, hatred and fear of men, and feelings of guilt. A physician's responsibility to a rape victim is to make sure she is protected prophylactically against pregnancy, to carefully record medical evidence of the rape, and to provide for counseling. Although tests for venereal disease immediately following a rape could not yet be positive as a result of the rape and although the testing itself can be emotionally harmful, for medicolegal reasons these tests should be performed immediately to document absence of disease in the victim at the time of the rape. In one study of sexual offenders, the most common type of offender was a man who randomly selected unknown victims and found violence to be necessary for sexual fulfillment.

**143-147. The answers are: 143-A, 144-E, 145-D, 146-C, 147-B.** *(Romney, ed 2. pp 49-52.)* With increasing frequency physicians are called upon to become involved in the bioethical considerations of the circumstances surrounding death. The physician should be familiar with the terms used in order to better understand the debates on the moral and philosophical issues of this matter. **Negative or passive euthanasia** is the deliberate withholding or nonadministration of an agent without which the occurrence of death and perhaps its time of occurrence are reasonably foreseeable, whether it is preventable or not. **Positive or active euthanasia** is described as an act in which a person, other than the person dying, administers an agent that induces an intentional "good" death. **Facilitated suicide**

is the induction of one's own death after someone else has purposefully made available the agent of death. The dying person may then exercise choice to use or not use the means of death made easily available to her or him. **Suicide** is the induction of one's own death by the administration of a lethal agent not intentionally procured by someone else.

# Contraception, Abortion, and Sterilization

**DIRECTIONS**: Each question below contains five suggested answers. Choose the **one best** response to each question.

148. The use of combined birth-control pills is contraindicated in women who have all of the following EXCEPT

(A) sickle cell anemia
(B) diabetes
(C) chronic cholestatic liver disease
(D) atrial fibrillation
(E) history of thromboemboli

149. Atypical adenomatous hyperplasia of the cervix has been associated with the use of oral contraceptives. Which of the following statements about this disorder is true?

(A) It develops within 3 months of initiation of oral contraception
(B) If left untreated, it usually progresses to a frankly malignant disease
(C) Mitotic figures are histologically common
(D) Lesions usually are friable and prone to bleeding
(E) Only the cells of endocervical glands are affected

150. The manufacture of ethinyl estradiol was an important breakthrough in the development of oral contraceptives, because the agent was discovered to be

(A) an especially effective estrogen
(B) orally active
(C) less potent and therefore better tolerated than diethylstilbestrol
(D) the endogenously active form of estrogen
(E) an estrogen with a unique action on the hypothalamus

151. Birth-control pills have been associated with hepatic adenomas. Most of these tumors are

(A) benign
(B) hormone producing
(C) diabetogenic
(D) associated with thromboembolism
(E) associated with urinary tract infections

152. The **pregnancy rate**, a term frequently used to describe the effectiveness of a given contraceptive technique, is defined as the

(A) percentage of pregnancies resulting from a single coital exposure
(B) percentage of pregnancies resulting from multiple coital exposures
(C) number of pregnancies occurring per 100 woman-years of use
(D) number of live births per 1000 women of reproductive age
(E) number of live births per 1000 people

153. The major cause of oral-contraceptive failure resulting in an unplanned pregnancy is

(A) breakthrough ovulation at mid-cycle
(B) frequency of intercourse
(C) incorrect use of oral-contraceptive pills
(D) gastrointestinal malabsorption
(E) development of antibodies

154. A pregnancy of approximately 10 weeks gestation is confirmed in a 30-year-old woman (gravida 5, para 4) with an intrauterine device (IUD) in place. The patient expresses a strong desire for the pregnancy to be continued. On examination the strings of the IUD are protruding from the cervical os. The most appropriate course of action would be to

(A) leave the IUD in place without any other treatment
(B) leave the IUD in place and continue prophylactic antibiotics throughout pregnancy
(C) remove the IUD immediately
(D) terminate the pregnancy because of the near certain risk of infection, abortion, or both
(E) perform laparoscopy to rule out an ectopic pregnancy

**DIRECTIONS:** Each question below contains four suggested answers of which **one** or **more** is correct. Choose the answer:

| A | if | 1, 2, and 3 | are correct |
|---|---|---|---|
| B | if | 1 and 3 | are correct |
| C | if | 2 and 4 | are correct |
| D | if | 4 | is correct |
| E | if | 1, 2, 3, and 4 | are correct |

155. Progestational agents in birth-control pills have which of the following actions?

(1) Inhibition of secretion of hypothalamic releasing factor
(2) Endometrial decidualization
(3) Thickening of cervical mucus
(4) Prevention of irregular menses

156. A 26-year-old woman, who comes to your office to renew her supply of birth-control pills, has mild hypertension, truncal obesity, and acne. Laboratory evaluation reveals that her serum levels of free cortisol are increased; this increase could be due to which of the following reasons?

(1) Cushing's disease
(2) Displacement of cortisol from transcortin by progesterone
(3) Estrogen-related interference of the liver's ability to metabolize cortisol
(4) An increase in ACTH production caused by ingestion of birth-control pills

157. Coitus interruptus (withdrawal) often fails as a method of birth control, because

(1) prostatic secretions containing sperm are released during the excitement and plateau phases of sex response
(2) pelvic thrusting becomes involuntary before ejaculation occurs
(3) many men start ejaculating before they realize it
(4) Cowper's gland secretions often contain sperm

158. The theoretical effectiveness of a given contraceptive is affected by

(1) patient motivation
(2) its relationship to the act of coitus
(3) its ease of use
(4) its antifertility action

159. The insertion of an IUD would be contraindicated in a 24-year-old woman under which of the following conditions?

(1) A recent, unexplained, abnormal Papanicolaou (Pap) smear
(2) The absence of a previous pregnancy
(3) Previously treated episodes of pelvic inflammatory disease
(4) The presence of menses

160. A young woman is seen immediately after being raped on day 14 of a usually regular 28-day cycle. Accepted methods of preventing an unwanted pregnancy include

(1) diethylstilbestrol, 25 mg twice a day for 5 days
(2) initiation of oral contraceptives
(3) insertion of an IUD
(4) intramuscular medroxyprogesterone acetate, 150 mg

161. In patients taking combination-type birth-control pills, altered metabolic functions may include

(1) a decrease in glucose tolerance
(2) an increase in binding globulins
(3) an increase in sodium sulfobromophthalein (Bromsulphalein) retention
(4) an increase in triglycerides

162. A woman who is 12 weeks pregnant undergoes an outpatient suction abortion. She returns 3 days later with a temperature of 39.2°C (102.5°F), lower abdominal cramps, and vaginal bleeding. The uterus is boggy on examination. Appropriate therapy should include

(1) culture and Gram stain of the endocervix
(2) culture of venous blood
(3) antibiotic therapy
(4) uterine curettage

163. Termination of pregnancy (intentional abortion) in the first trimester may be

(1) followed by Rh sensitization
(2) performed without dilating the cervix
(3) performed by either sharp or suction curettage
(4) regulated by state law

164. Midtrimester intentional abortion by instillation of hypertonic saline into the amniotic cavity may be

(1) regulated by state law
(2) followed by Rh sensitization
(3) followed by disseminated intravascular coagulation
(4) followed by permanent hypertension

165. True statements regarding operative procedures for sterilization include which of the following?

(1) They can be performed immediately postpartum
(2) They have become the most common method of contraception for white couples between 20 and 40 years of age in the United States
(3) They can be considered effective immediately in females (bilateral tubal ligation)
(4) They can be considered effective immediately in males (vasectomy)

| SUMMARY OF DIRECTIONS | | | | |
|---|---|---|---|---|
| A | B | C | D | E |
| 1, 2, 3 only | 1, 3 only | 2, 4 only | 4 only | All are correct |

166. Comparisons between unmarried women and married women reveal that

(1) married women have a higher incidence of phobias than unmarried women
(2) married women have a lower incidence of depression than unmarried women
(3) married women have a higher incidence of hypochondriasis than unmarried women
(4) married women are less apt to be dissatisfied with their jobs than unmarried women

167. Compliance with a therapeutic program is related to a patient's

(1) understanding of the necessity of therapy
(2) relationship with the physician
(3) financial ability to carry out the program
(4) motivation to carry out the therapeutic plan

Contraception, Abortion, and Sterilization 71

DIRECTIONS: The groups of questions below consist of lettered choices followed by several numbered items. For each numbered item select the **one** lettered choice with which it is **most** closely associated. Each lettered choice may be used once, more than once, or not at all.

Questions 168-173

For each situation listed below, select the most appropriate response.

(A) Stop pills and resume after 7 days
(B) Continue pills as usual
(C) Continue pills and use an additional form of contraception
(D) Take an additional pill
(E) Stop pills and seek a medical examination

168. Nausea during first cycle of pills

169. No menses during 7 days following 21-day cycle of correct use

170. Forgot pill 1 day

171. Forgot pill 10 continuous days

172. Light bleeding at midcycle during first month on pill

173. Hemoptysis

Questions 174-178

For each description that follows, select the pharmacological agent with which it is most likely to be associated.

(A) Testosterone
(B) Mestranol
(C) Norethindrone
(D) Clomiphene
(E) Medroxyprogesterone acetate

174. A progestin commonly used in oral contraceptives

175. An orally active estrogen

176. Commercially marketed as Depo-Provera

177. An antiestrogenic agent

178. An agent that causes an increase in endogenous estrogen

## Questions 179-185

The pregnancy rate in a sexually active population not using contraception is approximately 80 pregnancies. For each of the following contraceptive techniques, select the most appropriate pregnancy rate based on use effectiveness.

(A) 80
(B) 15
(C) 7
(D) 2
(E) Less than 1

179. Rhythm method

180. Intrauterine contraceptive device (IUD)

181. Vaginal diaphragm

182. Postcoital douche

183. Oral contraceptives (birth-control pills)

184. Withdrawal

185. Condoms

## Questions 186-190

For each description that follows, select the type of abortion with which it is most commonly associated.

(A) Spontaneous abortion
(B) Threatened abortion
(C) Habitual abortion
(D) Missed abortion
(E) Medical therapeutic abortion

186. Occurs in 20 percent of all pregnancies

187. Occurs in 10 percent of all pregnancies

188. Blighted ovum is responsible for 50 percent

189. May be associated with coagulation defect

190. Not anticipated with the first pregnancy

# Contraception, Abortion, and Sterilization
# Answers

**148. The answer is B.** *(Speroff, ed 2. pp 290-300.)* Sickle cell anemia, atrial fibrillation, and previous pulmonary embolus are contraindications to the use of birth-control pills, because clotting is enhanced by increased levels of fibrinogen. It also has been shown that oral contraceptives markedly increase cholestasis in women who are sensitive to this effect of estrogen; this cholestasis resembles cholestatic jaundice of pregnancy. Although diabetes might be made worse in diabetic women taking birth-control pills, the value of effective contraception may outweigh the pills' negative effects; for these women, an increase in their insulin dose may be a satisfactory precaution. The use of oral contraceptives, however, is not recommended for diabetic women who do not take insulin but who would require it once oral contraceptive therapy has begun.

**149. The answer is D.** *(Green, ed 3. p 244.)* Atypical adenomatous hyperplasia of the cervix associated with oral contraceptives is most significant because it often is confused with adenocarcinoma of the cervix. Because of the polypoid, friable nature of the lesions, affected women often present with contact bleeding. The lesions are benign, and histological examination shows gland-cell and reserve-cell hyperplasia without any of the characteristics, such as abundance of mitotic figures, of malignancy. Atypical adenomatous hyperplasia of the cervix most commonly develops in women who have used oral contraceptives for several years.

**150. The answer is B.** *(Speroff, ed 2. pp 283-284.)* An ethinyl group added at the 17 position makes ethinyl estradiol a very potent, orally active estrogen. Until this discovery in 1938, no orally effective estrogen had been manufactured. The effects of ethinyl estradiol on the hypothalamus and peripheral receptors are not different from other estrogens. Its contraceptive properties are therefore similar to other estrogens. The contraceptive properties of ethinyl estradiol are not significantly different from other estrogens. Ethinyl estradiol is up to 25 times as potent as diethylstilbestrol.

**151. The answer is A.** *(Wynn, ed 2. p 233.)* Focal nodular hyperplasia of the liver and hepatic adenomas are unusual complications of birth-control pills. Even though most pill-induced hepatic adenomas are benign, they have been associated with rupture and serious hemorrhage. Birth-control pills on occasion may be associated with such diverse complications as urinary tract infection, thromboembolism, altered carbohydrate metabolism, and hormonal effects. These changes are ascribed to the pills and are not signs of an hepatic tumor.

**152. The answer is C.** *(Wynn, ed 2. p 226.)* The pregnancy rate is expressed by the following formula:

$$\text{Pregnancy rate} = \frac{\text{Number of pregnancies} \times 1200}{\text{Number of women observed} \times \text{months of exposure}}$$

In other words, the pregnancy rate is the number of pregnancies per 100 woman-years of use. The fertility rate is defined as the number of live births per 1000 women 15 to 44 years of age. The birth rate is defined as the number of births per 1000 population.

**153. The answer is C.** *(Wynn, ed 2. p 235.)* The pregnancy rate with birth-control pills, based on theoretical effectiveness, is 0.1 percent. However, the effectiveness in actual use is 0.7 percent. This increase is due to incorrect use of the pills. Breakthrough ovulation on combination birth-control pills is thought to be a very rare occurrence. The effectiveness of the pills is not related to sexual frequency, gastrointestinal disturbances, or the development of antibodies.

**154. The answer is C.** *(Wynn, ed 2. p 231.)* Although there is an increased risk of spontaneous abortion, and a small risk of infection, an intrauterine pregnancy can occur and continue successfully to term with an intrauterine device (IUD) in place. However, if the patient wishes to keep the pregnancy and if the strings are visible, the IUD should be removed in an attempt to reduce the risk of infection, abortion, or both. Although the percentage of ectopic pregnancies may be increased, the majority of pregnancies occurring with an IUD are intrauterine. Therefore, in the absence of signs and symptoms suggestive of an ectopic pregnancy, laparoscopy is not indicated.

**155. The answer is A (1, 2, 3).** *(Speroff, ed 2. p 288.)* Progestational agents in oral contraceptives work by a negative feedback mechanism to inhibit the secretion of hypothalamic releasing factor and, as a result, prevent ovulation. They also cause decidualization and atrophy of the endometrium, hence making implantation impossible. In addition, cervical mucus, which at ovulation is thin and watery, is changed by the influence of progestational agents to a tenacious com-

Contraception, Abortion, and Sterilization 75

pound that severely limits sperm motility; and some evidence indicates that they may change ovum and sperm migration patterns within the reproductive system. Progestins do not prevent irregular bleeding. Estrogen in birth-control pills enhances the negative feedback of the progestins and stabilizes the endometrium to prevent irregular menses.

**156.** The answer is A (1, 2, 3). *(Speroff, ed 2. pp 292-293.)* The clinical symptoms and increased free cortisol levels of the woman described in the question suggest Cushing's disease. Her elevated cortisol levels also could be due to certain metabolical effects of birth-control pills. It was once believed that the pill increased the transcortin level but not the free cortisol level; however, the free cortisol level may in fact increase because of displacement of free cortisol from transcortin by progesterone. The high levels of estrogen in women taking birth-control pills can hinder the liver's ability to metabolize cortisol, resulting in higher-than-normal cortisol levels. If the pill has any effect on pituitary production of ACTH, it is a suppressive one.

**157.** The answer is C (2, 4). *(Masters, 1966. pp 293, 298.)* Cowper's gland secretions, released in late plateau phase, are thought to contain sperm. Prostatic secretions probably do not contribute to this pre-ejaculatory emission. At the very end of the plateau phase, voluntary pelvic thrusting can become involuntary, therefore making withdrawal of the penis difficult. For 2 or 3 seconds before ejaculation, prostatic secretions fill the prostatic urethra, resulting in a feeling that the ejaculation is coming ("ejaculatory inevitability").

**158.** The answer is D (4). *(Wynn, ed 2. p 226.)* The theoretical effectiveness is the antifertility effectiveness of the contraceptive observed under optimal conditions, that is, when used properly and regularly. Use effectiveness, on the other hand, describes the actual effectiveness observed under realistic conditions. Use effectiveness is therefore influenced by such factors as cost, convenience of use, relationship to coitus, and the requirement for repeated patient motivation.

**159.** The answer is A (1, 2, 3). *(Wynn, ed 2. pp 230-231.)* Insertion of an IUD in the face of an unexplained abnormal Pap smear may interfere with diagnosis and also conceivably disseminate abnormal cells. Bacterial contamination associated with insertion into a patient whose local host defenses are impaired by tissues damaged from previous pelvic inflammatory disease could result in acute reinfection. In nulligravid patients, the risk of sterility resulting from complications of an IUD does not absolutely contraindicate its use; however, such risk should be explained in detail to the patient in order that other equally effective methods of contraception can be explored. Insertion of an IUD during menses eases the insertion and also gives added assurance against placement into a pregnant uterus.

**160. The answer is B (1, 3).** *(Mishell, pp 534-535. Wynn, ed 2. pp 238-239.)* While there is no universally accepted method of postcoital contraception, the Food and Drug Administration has approved diethylstilbestrol (DES) 25 mg twice daily for 5 days for use as a "morning after pill." An antiemetic may be given in conjunction with DES to minimize the associated nausea and vomiting. While one study has shown that a high dosage of birth control pills (two per day for 10 days, 12 hours apart) will prevent fertilization, this is not a widely used method. A normal dosage of birth control pills would not be effective. Insertion of an IUD will prevent implantation if fertilization should occur. Many clinicians feel all forms of postcoital contraception incur unwarranted risk of side effects to the majority of patients, while an early termination of pregnancy or menstrual extraction may be offered to those few patients requiring it. Injectable progesterone has not been shown to prevent contraception during a cycle in which ovulation may have already occurred.

**161. The answer is E (all).** *(Wynn, ed 2. p 233.)* Combination-type oral contraceptives are potent systemic steroids that may cause many detectable alterations in metabolic function, such as increases in binding globulins, Bromsulphalein retention, triglycerides, and total phospholipids, and a decrease in glucose tolerance. Thus, the benefits of birth-control pills must be weighed carefully against the added risks in patients with diabetes, cardiovascular disease, or liver disease.

**162. The answer is E (all).** *(Monif, pp 278-280.)* Culture and Gram stain of the endocervix are important in directing antibiotic therapy for women who have had septic abortions. Blood cultures also can be very helpful, because they are positive in 30 to 50 percent of patients who have an abortion-related infection. Broad-spectrum antibiotic therapy is, of course, indicated. Moreover, in a woman who has a fever, cramps, and vaginal bleeding following an abortion, retention of conception products must be suspected, and curettage should be performed.

**163. The answer is A (1, 2, 3).** *(Wynn, ed 2. pp 244-249.)* Significant fetomaternal transfusion may occur following first trimester abortions. Therefore, Rh-immune globulin should be administered to Rh-negative women whenever the products of conception may be Rh positive. A 1973 United States Supreme Court ruling specifically prohibits state regulation of abortions performed in the first trimester. In early pregnancy a small suction catheter (about 6 mm) can often be inserted and the pregnancy successfully terminated without dilating the cervix. Although suction curettage may be associated with slightly fewer complications, especially in larger uteri, than sharp curettage, either technique is acceptable.

Contraception, Abortion, and Sterilization 77

**164. The answer is A (1, 2, 3).** *(Wynn, ed 2. pp 244-249.)* Saline abortions performed in the midtrimester may be followed by significant fetomaternal transfusion. $Rh_O$ immunoglobulin (RhoGAM) should therefore be administered to Rh-negative patients under the same conditions as with a full-term pregnancy. Although state law may not prohibit midtrimester abortions, it may regulate their performance to protect maternal health. Although they are infrequent, many serious complications may follow a saline abortion. Among these are encephalopathy, hypernatremia, hemoglobinuria, cardiac arrest, tissue necrosis, and disseminated intravascular coagulation. Although acute cardiovascular reactions, including hypertension, do occur, they are not permanent.

**165. The answer is A (1, 2, 3).** *(Wynn, ed 2. pp 240-243.)* Sterilization has become the most commonly utilized method of contraception in the United States for white couples between 20 and 40 years of age. In an otherwise uncomplicated pregnancy, a tubal ligation can, if desired, be performed in the immediate postpartum period. Unless the woman has already conceived at the time of the procedure, the contraceptive effect is immediate. Vasectomy in the male, however, should not be considered effective until an examination of the ejaculate is sperm free on two successive occasions.

**166. The answer is B (1, 3).** *(Romney, ed 2. pp 861-863.)* At least 40 percent of marriages end in divorce, and in most cases it is the wife, not the husband, who considers the marriage an unhappy one. Psychological and physical anxieties are both more common among married women than among married men. However, in a comparison of married and unmarried women, unmarried women were found to be far less subject to anxiety, depression, hypochondriasis, and job dissatisfaction. Unmarried women also were found to be healthier than unmarried men, as well as to have higher educational levels and higher average incomes.

**167. The answer is E (all).** *(Ryan, pp 255-256.)* A patient's compliance with various therapeutic regimens is of prime importance in the care of ambulatory patients. A good relationship with the physician, an understanding of the necessity of therapy, and the financial and motivational abilities to carry out the therapy are important factors in compliance and should be assessed at the conclusion of each visit. At that time it is appropriate to expand the patient's understanding of the disease process to improve motivation.

**168-173. The answers are: 168-B, 169-B, 170-D, 171-C, 172-B, 173-E.** *(Wynn, ed 2. pp 233-236.)* Common side effects of birth-control pills include nausea, breakthrough bleeding, bloating, and leg cramps. If these side effects are experienced in the first two or three cycles of pills, when they are most common, the pills may be safely continued as these effects usually remit spontaneously.

On occasion, following correct use of a full cycle of pills, withdrawal bleeding may fail to occur (silent menses). Pregnancy is a very unlikely explanation for this event; therefore, pills should be resumed as usual (after 7 days) just as if bleeding had occurred. However, if a second consecutive period has been missed, pregnancy should be more seriously considered and ruled out by a pregnancy test, medical examination, or both.

Women occasionally forget to take pills; however, when only a single pill has been omitted, it can be taken immediately in addition to the usual pill at the usual time. This single-pill omission is associated with little if any loss in effectiveness. If three or more pills are omitted, the pills should be resumed as usual, but an additional contraceptive method (e.g., condoms) should be used through one full cycle.

Although most side effects caused by birth-control pills can be considered minor, serious side effects do sometimes occur. A painful swollen calf may signal thrombophlebitis. Hemoptysis may signal pulmonary embolism. Either of these circumstances should be considered a medical emergency, and immediate medical attention should be sought.

**174-178. The answers are: 174-C, 175-B, 176-E, 177-D, 178-D.** *(Speroff, ed 2. pp 284-287, 375-377.)* Ethinyl estradiol and mestranol are the two active synthetic estrogens used in birth-control pills (mestranol is employed more commonly than ethinyl estradiol). An ethinyl group at the 17 position makes these estrogens orally active.

By removing the 19 carbon from testosterone, a nontestosterone, orally active progestational agent (a 19-nortestosterone) is obtained. Norethindrone is the most commonly used progestational agent of this type in birth-control pills.

The progestational agent medroxyprogesterone acetate (Depo-Provera), along with chlormadinone, has been noted to produce benign breast tumors in beagle puppies; when estrogens were administered at the same time, however, this effect could not be reproduced.

Clomiphene is a nonsteroidal antiestrogenic agent. By inhibiting hypothalamic regulation of estrogen production, causing estrogen levels to increase, clomiphene can promote ovulation in certain groups of anovulatory women.

# Contraception, Abortion, and Sterilization 79

**179-185. The answers are: 179-B, 180-D, 181-C, 182-A, 183-E, 184-B, 185-C.** *(Wynn, ed 2. pp 226-235.)* Contraceptive effectiveness is frequently described in terms of the pregnancy associated with its use:

$$\text{Pregnancy rate} = \frac{\text{Number of pregnancies} \times 1200}{\text{Number of women observed} \times \text{months of exposure}}$$

This formula expresses the number of pregnancies to be expected with 100 woman-years of use.

The effectiveness of the rhythm method is influenced by the woman's ability to predict the time of ovulation from the regularity of her menses. It is also influenced by the woman's motivation to successfully abstain from intercourse during the 10 days around suspected ovulation. These menstrual and ovulatory irregularities and lapses in the woman's motivation account for a pregnancy rate of 15 with the rhythm method.

In contrast to the rhythm method, the IUD requires little or no action on the part of the woman. For this reason the device's actual use effectiveness approaches its maximal theoretical effectiveness and a pregnancy rate of 2.

The vaginal diaphragm and the condom are barrier contraceptives in that for each act of sexual intercourse they pose a barrier between the sperm ejaculate and the endocervical canal. In theory both can be very effective. However, both require recurrent motivation for application with each act of intercourse. Lapses in motivation are not uncommon, and there is a pregnancy rate of 7 for each of these two methods.

The pregnancy rate with postcoital douching is almost the same as that for unprotected intercourse (80). This lack of effectiveness is readily explained by the extremely rapid progression of motile sperm into the endocervical canal, coupled with the failure of a vaginal douche to reach this area.

Combined oral contraceptive birth-control pills are clearly the most effective reversible contraceptive currently available. With correct use many studies report a contraceptive effectiveness that approaches 100 percent (pregnancy rate $<0.1$). This extreme effectiveness is best explained by its multiplicity of actions, that is, suppression of ovulation, hostility of the cervical mucus to sperm penetration, and hostility of atrophic endometrium to the implantation of a conceptus.

Withdrawal, also termed coitus interruptus, is a contraceptive technique in common use throughout the world. It is associated with a pregnancy rate of 15. Pregnancies with this technique are readily explained by the frequent occurrence of an involuntary pre-ejaculatory dribble and also by the ability of sperm to occasionally gain entrance to the vagina when deposited on the external genitalia.

**186-190. The answers are: 186-B, 187-A, 188-A, 189-D, 190-C.** *(Pritchard, ed 16. pp 588-597.)* Abortion is defined as a pregnancy that terminates before the fetus is sufficiently developed to survive. Many different types of abortion have been identified.

Threatened abortion signified by vaginal bleeding in early pregnancy occurs in about 20 percent of all pregnancies; in about 50 percent of these, the cause is implantation of a normal ovum. In these cases of implantation bleeding, the bleeding would be expected to cease and the pregnancy to continue in a normal fashion. In the other 50 percent of threatened abortions (10 percent of all pregnancies) the bleeding will continue and spontaneous abortion will follow. A blighted ovum is the most common cause (50 percent) for spontaneous abortion.

Occasionally the products of conception will die, yet spontaneous abortion does not ensue. This prolonged retention of a dead fetus in the first half of pregnancy is termed a missed abortion. On rare occasions this prolonged retention of dead tissue can be associated with disseminated intravascular coagulation, a serious coagulation disorder.

Habitual abortion is generally considered to be three or more consecutive spontaneous abortions. Although there are many causes for this disorder, it is probably a chance phenomenon most of the time.

# NORMAL PREGNANCY

# The Fetus, Placenta, and Newborn

DIRECTIONS: Each question below contains five suggested answers. Choose the one best response to each question.

191. During labor, deceleration of the fetal heart rate correlates most closely with which of the following fetal values?
(A) Arterial pH
(B) Arterial $P_{O_2}$
(C) Arterial $P_{CO_2}$
(D) Central venous pressure
(E) Venous potassium levels

192. A 28-year-old primigravid woman first registers for prenatal care at 36 weeks gestation. A tuberculin skin (PPD) test is positive. The woman states that she has never had a PPD test before. A chest x-ray is ordered, but the woman does not keep her appointment and, in fact, does not return to the hospital until labor has begun at 41 weeks. A chest x-ray at this time reveals minimal tuberculous changes. The woman is kept in the hospital until all of the cultures for acid-fast bacilli are reported to be negative. She is started on isoniazid (INH) chemotherapy. Appropriate treatment of the neonate would include
(A) isolation from the mother for 3 to 6 weeks
(B) administration of INH
(C) vaccination with BCG vaccine
(D) a PPD test every 3 to 4 months
(E) none of the above

193. At term, a pregnant woman has herpesvirus hominis (herpes simplex) type 2 lesions on her vulva and vagina. What is the chance that her infant will develop an infection after delivery?
(A) 0.5 percent
(B) 1 percent
(C) 5 percent
(D) 30 percent
(E) 75 percent

194. All of the following drugs can cross the placenta easily EXCEPT
(A) digoxin
(B) phenobarbital
(C) heparin
(D) mepivacaine
(E) tetracycline

195. Cytomegalovirus, which can cause severe intrauterine infection, can be recovered from the cervices of approximately what percentage of women in the United States?
(A) 0.005 percent
(B) 0.05 percent
(C) 0.5 percent
(D) 5 percent
(E) 50 percent

196. A syndrome of multiple congenital anomalies, including microcephaly, cardiac anomalies, and growth retardation, has been described in children of women who are heavy users of

(A) amphetamines
(B) barbiturates
(C) heroin
(D) methadone
(E) ethyl alcohol

197. Epidemiological or clinical studies support all of the following statements concerning the effects of cigarette smoking during pregnancy EXCEPT that

(A) there is a reduction in birth weight of the offspring of smokers when compared to matched controls
(B) the incidence of premature labor is not statistically significant in women who smoke
(C) the incidence of pregnancy-induced hypertension is increased in women who smoke
(D) the effects of smoking are directly proportional to the number of cigarettes smoked
(E) the number of cigarettes smoked daily after the third month of gestation is more important than the number smoked before that time

198. The relationship between fetal, placental, and maternal endocrine systems is characterized by

(A) identical enzymatic capabilities
(B) the addition of sulfate radicals in the placental compartment
(C) placental conversion of C-21 compounds to C-19 compounds
(D) the principal conversion of dehydroepiandrosterone sulfate to estrogens by the maternal compartment
(E) none of the above

199. At 20 weeks gestation, the crown-rump length of the fetus is approximately

(A) 9 cm
(B) 12 cm
(C) 14 cm
(D) 16 cm
(E) 19 cm

200. The normal umbilical cord contains which of the following systems of blood vessels?

(A) One artery and one vein
(B) One artery and two veins
(C) Two arteries and one vein
(D) Two arteries and two veins
(E) None of the above

**DIRECTIONS**: Each question below contains four suggested answers of which **one** or **more** is correct. Choose the answer:

| | | | |
|---|---|---|---|
| A | if | 1, 2, and 3 | are correct |
| B | if | 1 and 3 | are correct |
| C | if | 2 and 4 | are correct |
| D | if | 4 | is correct |
| E | if | 1, 2, 3, and 4 | are correct |

201. A full-term infant is found to have a heart rate less than 100 beats per minute at 1 minute after birth. The infant does not cry and has central cyanosis, slow and irregular respiration, and some flexion of the extremities. The obstetrician should

(1) start immediate resuscitation
(2) give the infant a 1-minute Apgar score of 3
(3) call for pediatric consultation
(4) assume that adequate ventilation will correct the respiratory depression

202. True statements about the twin-twin transfusion syndrome include which of the following?

(1) The donor twin develops hydramnios more often than the recipient twin
(2) Gross differences may be observed between donor and recipient placentas
(3) The donor twin usually suffers from a hemolytic anemia
(4) The recipient twin can develop widespread thromboses

203. An infant is likely to be compromised as a result of vaginal delivery that is accompanied by which of the following conditions?

(1) Prolapse of the umbilical cord
(2) Shoulder presentation
(3) Persistent brow presentation
(4) Persistent occiput posterior position

204. The human placenta produces which of the following hormones?

(1) Gonadotropin
(2) Somatomammotropin
(3) Progesterone
(4) Hydrocortisone

205. Chorioangiomas can be described by which of the following statements?

(1) They affect more than 5 percent of placentas
(2) They often are associated with anomalous cord insertions
(3) They often are associated with cords containing only two vessels
(4) They are the most common tumors of the placenta

206. True statements about placental infarcts include which of the following?
(1) They result from thrombosis of the decidual spiral arterioles
(2) They are present in approximately 5 to 20 percent of all third-trimester deliveries
(3) They occur twice as frequently in white women as in black women
(4) They are frequently associated with pre-eclampsia and essential hypertension

207. Substances that cross the placenta poorly or not at all include
(1) thyroxine
(2) long-acting thyroid stimulator
(3) thyroid-stimulating hormone
(4) propylthiouracil

208. True statements describing toxoplasmosis in a pregnant woman include which of the following?
(1) It can be acquired by eating infected raw meat
(2) It occurs in 1 in every 2000 to 2500 pregnancies
(3) Infection in early pregnancy may lead to abortion
(4) Transplacental infection of the fetus is highly unlikely

209. True statements about a pregnant woman who has phenylketonuria include which of the following?
(1) If her offspring are mentally retarded, they almost certainly have phenylketonuria
(2) A maternal diet low in phenylalanine and instituted by the third trimester can block development of mental retardation in the child
(3) Recommending an abortion is rarely justified
(4) If the maternal diet is unrestricted, the risk of having a mentally retarded child is nearly 100 percent

210. Maternal diabetes mellitus is associated with which of the following symptoms in the fetus or neonate?
(1) Macrosomia in the fetus
(2) Delayed pulmonic maturity in the fetus
(3) Hypoglycemia in the newborn
(4) Hypocalcemia in the newborn

211. Situations that increase the risk of morbidity or mortality for the fetus of a diabetic mother include
(1) maternal ketoacidosis
(2) maternal ketonuria in the absence of diabetic ketoacidosis
(3) maternal hyperglycemia
(4) maternal hypoglycemia

## SUMMARY OF DIRECTIONS

| A | B | C | D | E |
|---|---|---|---|---|
| 1, 2, 3 only | 1, 3 only | 2, 4 only | 4 only | All are correct |

212. Signs of fetal postmaturity that may be noted prior to delivery include

(1) oligohydramnios
(2) maternal edema
(3) meconium-stained amniotic fluid
(4) maternal weight loss

213. Severe fetal or neonatal infection can result from maternal infection near term by which of the following viruses?

(1) Group B coxsackievirus
(2) Rubella virus
(3) Chickenpox virus
(4) Herpesvirus hominis, type 2

214. Substances that are normally found in higher concentrations in maternal blood than in fetal or umbilical cord blood include

(1) immunoglobulin G (IgG)
(2) immunoglobulin M (IgM)
(3) gamma chains of hemoglobin
(4) fibrinogen

215. True statements about the lecithin-to-sphingomyelin ratio include which of the following?

(1) It can reflect total muscle mass of the fetus
(2) It rises later than normal if toxemia of pregnancy has developed
(3) It rises earlier than normal if erythroblastosis fetalis has developed
(4) It can reflect fetal surfactant production

216. Acute obstruction of the umbilical circulation has been found experimentally to provoke which of the following responses?

(1) A rapid fall in fetal central venous pressure
(2) An almost immediate fall in fetal heart rate
(3) A rapidly mediated humoral effect on the fetal heart
(4) A rapidly mediated response by the fetal heart that can be affected by cutting the vagi

217. The twin-twin transfusion syndrome can be associated with which of the following?

(1) Diamniotic, monochorionic placentas
(2) Twins of opposite sex
(3) Monoamniotic, monochorionic placentas
(4) Fused diamniotic, dichorionic placentas

218. True statements about monozygotic twinning include which of the following?

(1) It tends to run in families
(2) It frequently is associated with pregnancies induced by clomiphene citrate
(3) It is more common than dizygotic twinning
(4) It occurs in approximately 1 pregnancy in 250

**DIRECTIONS:** The group of questions below consists of lettered choices followed by several numbered items. For each numbered item select the **one** lettered choice with which it is **most** closely associated. Each lettered choice may be used once, more than once, or not at all.

**Questions 219-222**

For each of the following substances, choose the mechanism of transplacental transport most likely to be employed.

(A) Simple diffusion
(B) Facilitated diffusion
(C) Active transport
(D) Pinocytosis
(E) None of the above

219. Carbon dioxide

220. Iron

221. Oxygen

222. Glucose

# The Fetus, Placenta, and Newborn Answers

**191. The answer is B.** *(Aladjem, ed 2. pp 341-344.)* Deceleration of the fetal heart rate is related to hypoxia. Although fetal hypoxia also leads to a metabolic acidosis, which is reflected by a low arterial pH and increased base deficits, deceleration of the fetal heart rate occurs before development of the acidosis.

**192. The answer is C.** *(Burrow, pp 578-579.)* The mother described in the question would be said to have inactive, not previously treated tuberculosis. The chance of reactivation of the disease is 1 to 4.5 percent a year. Isoniazid (INH) should be used preventively in the mother and continued for a year. If the mother has inactive disease that has been treated, the baby need not be treated. If the mother has inactive disease and is currently being treated, it normally would be permissible for her to have contact with the baby, who again need not be treated. However, the patient described presents a special problem. Because she has given evidence of being unreliable, her ability to take INH at the prescribed dosage for the prescribed time is suspect. Placing the baby on preventive INH therapy can endanger the child, if the mother fails to administer the drug faithfully. Thus, the safest course would be to vaccinate the baby with BCG vaccine, an immunizing agent against tuberculosis consisting of a culture of the Calmette-Guérin bacillus.

**193. The answer is D.** *(Nahmias, Am J Obstet Gynecol 110:825, 1971.)* Herpesvirus hominis type 2 infection is highly contagious and develops in 20 to at least 40 percent of all neonates delivered vaginally from women who have herpetic vulvovaginitis. These neonatal infections are usually fulminant and are associated with a mortality rate of more than 60 percent. In addition, neurological or ocular disease affects most of the survivors.

**194. The answer is C.** *(Adamsons, Am J Obstet Gynecol 96:437, 1966.)* Because of its large molecular size and strong electronegativity, heparin cannot cross tissue boundaries easily. Warfarin (Coumadin), on the other hand, easily crosses the placental barrier and thus can cause anticoagulation in a fetus. All of the other drugs listed in the question easily cross the placenta and can be recovered from fetal blood.

**195. The answer is D.** *(Monif, p 43.)* Cytomegalovirus is found in 3 to 6 percent of endocervical cultures of American women. However, unlike herpesvirus, the presence of cytomegalovirus in the cervix does not pose a major threat to the fetus passing through the genital canal. Cytomegalovirus can cause a severe intrauterine infection, however, if viremia results in a transplacental infection.

**196. The answer is E.** *(Burrow, pp 898-899.)* Chronic alcohol abuse, which can cause liver disease, folate deficiency, and many other disorders in a pregnant woman, also can lead to the development of congenital abnormalities in the child. The chief abnormalities associated with the fetal alcohol syndrome are microcephaly, growth retardation, and cardiac anomalies. Chronic abuse of alcohol also may be associated with an increased incidence of mental retardation in the children of affected women.

**197. The answer is C.** *(Burrow, p 901. Butler Br Med J 2:127-130, 1972. U.S. Department of Health, Education and Welfare, #(PHS) 79-50066:11-43, 1979.)* The incidence of pregnancy-induced hypertension seems to be decreased in women who smoke during pregnancy; this curious fact, which has yet to be explained, is supported by a number of epidemiological studies. Offspring of women who smoke more than five cigarettes daily from about the fourth month of pregnancy show decreases in birth weight of as much as 400 g when compared with matched controls.

The issue of premature delivery is a difficult one in that epidemiological studies reveal no overall downward shift in the distribution of gestational ages for infants of mothers who smoke; thus there appears to be a greater risk of true growth retardation rather than preterm delivery. However, there is a dose-related increase in the **proportion** of preterm babies born to women who smoke. These preterm deliveries account for a small proportion of total births so that the mean of gestational age distribution remains unchanged, yet these deliveries account for a large proportion of neonatal deaths. Therefore, while overall results show only a 0.02-week decrease in mean duration of pregnancy between smokers and nonsmokers, the rate of delivery before 38 weeks is $>7$ per 1000 births for nonsmokers, 92 per 1000 for light smokers, and 116 per 1000 for heavy smokers.

**198. The answer is E.** *(Burrow, p 912. Pritchard, ed 16. pp 147-164.)* The fetal, placental, and maternal compartments have very different enzymatic capacities. Conversion of C-21 to C-19 compounds can occur in the ovaries and the fetal adrenal glands, but not in the placenta. Fetal adrenals convert progesterone to dehydroepiandrosterone, to which a sulfate radical is added by the fetal liver. The placenta has the capacity to convert dehydroepiandrosterone sulfate to estrogens far more efficiently than the maternal compartment.

**199. The answer is D.** *(Pritchard, ed 16. p 174.)* If a fetus weighs less than 500 g or is less than 20 weeks gestational age at delivery, an abortion, as opposed to a birth, is usually recorded for purposes of perinatal statistics. When a birth weight has not been obtained, a crown-rump length of 16 cm indicates a gestational age of 20 weeks. However, at 500 g, a fetus is more likely to have attained at least 22 weeks gestation with a crown-rump length of approximately 19 cm.

**200. The answer is C.** *(Pritchard, ed 16. p 573.)* The normal umbilical cord contains two arteries and one vein. The absence of one umbilical artery is found in less than 1 percent of all infants. Although the significance of a missing umbilical artery is somewhat controversial, absence of the artery may indicate that other congenital anomalies also are present. Therefore, the obstetrician must verify the number of umbilical vessels and notify the pediatrician of any abnormality.

**201. The answer is A.** *(Pritchard, ed 16. pp 476-477.)* The assessment tool for infants known as the Apgar score is based on the infant's condition 1 minute and 5 minutes after birth. Heart rate, respiratory effort, muscle tone, reflex irritability, and body color are assessed. The maximum score is 10 (2 points per category), and the lowest score is 0. A perfect score indicates heart rate greater than 100 beats per minute, good respiratory effort, active motion, vigorous crying, and pink body color. Responses that are present but not optimal earn a score of 1 per category, while an absence of response gives no score. Apgar scores of 4 to 7 at 1 minute indicate mild respiratory depression; infants who score under 4 are severely depressed. Thus, a low 1-minute Apgar score indicates the need for immediate resuscitation, and a low 5-minute Apgar score indicates increased risk of morbidity and mortality. The infant presented in the question is severely depressed, and the physician should assume nothing regarding resuscitation.

**202. The answer is C (2, 4).** *(Benirschke, NY State J Med 61:4499, 1961.)* In the twin-twin transfusion syndrome, the donor twin is always anemic, due not to a hemolytic process but to the direct transfer of blood to the recipient twin. The recipient may suffer thromboses secondary to hypertransfusion and subsequent hemoconcentration. Although the donor placenta is usually pale and somewhat atrophied, that of the recipient is congested and enlarged. Hydramnios can develop in either twin but, because of circulatory overload, is more frequent in the recipient. Hydramnios when it occurs in the donor is due to congestive heart failure caused by severe anemia.

**203. The answer is A (1, 2, 3).** *(Pritchard, ed 16. pp 806-820.)* Shoulder presentation, either as a transverse or an oblique lie, presents significant problems when vaginal delivery of an affected infant is attempted, because the shoulder is arrested by the margins of the pelvic inlet. Similarly, persistent brow presentation compromises the infant because the resultant extensive molding deforms the head. The presence of a prolapsed umbilical cord is also associated with significant compromise of infants delivered vaginally, since the cord becomes compressed between the presenting part and the margin of the pelvic inlet. Persistent occiput posterior position does not significantly compromise an infant during the course of a normal vaginal delivery.

**204. The answer is A (1, 2, 3).** *(Pritchard, ed 16. pp 147-150, 162-164.)* The polypeptide hormones human chorionic gonadotropin (HCG) and human chorionic somatomammotropin (HCS) are produced by the syncytiotrophoblast of the human placenta. Because these hormones reflect placental rather than fetal integrity, the presence of HCG in the urine or blood may persist after fetal death (in the case of missed abortion) and even after spontaneous or therapeutic abortion. HCG is immunologically quite similar to pituitary luteinizing hormone (LH), the difference being in the amino-acid sequence of the beta subunit. This fact must be considered when interpreting results of pregnancy tests based on HCG bioassay, results of which are not always positive until 42 days gestation. The specific immunoassay for the beta subunit of HCG, on the other hand, may be positive even before a menstrual period is missed. Progesterone is made in large amounts by the placenta. There is no good evidence to support a placental role in the production of adrenocorticosteroids.

**205. The answer is D (4).** *(Aladjem, ed 2. p 284.)* Chorioangiomas are the most common placental tumor, occurring in approximately 1 percent of placentas. Despite attempts to correlate the presence of this tumor with hydramnios and fetal anomalies, no significant effect on fetal morbidity and mortality has been demonstrated, unless the size of the tumor is very great.

**206. The answer is E (all).** *(Aladjem, ed 2. p 286.)* Although the incidence of placental infarction in the United States is twice as high for white women as it is for black women, the perinatal mortality rate shows just the opposite relationship. Placental infarcts, which are caused by thrombosis of the decidual spiral arterioles, are present in up to 20 percent of all placentas at delivery. Diseases, such as essential hypertension and pre-eclampsia, that can cause the vascular changes associated with placental infarction may be more important in causing fetal compromise than the infarct itself.

**207. The answer is B (1, 3).** *(Burrow, pp 218-219, 226-236.)* Thyroxine crosses the placenta poorly, if at all. For this reason, a hyperthyroid mother does not transmit her hyperthyroidism to the fetus, and giving thyroid hormone to a hypothyroid mother will not raise fetal thyroxine levels significantly. Thyroid-stimulating hormone also does not cross to the fetus. On the other hand, propylthiouracil (PTU), an antithyroid drug, crosses easily and may suppress fetal thyroid function. Hyperthyroid women taking large doses of PTU therefore run the risk of having goitrous babies. Some clinicians, hoping to reverse the effect of PTU on the fetus, have given thyroxine to the mother; theoretically, however, this should not work, because the thyroid hormone should not get to the fetus. Long-acting thyroid stimulator (LATS) is present in many patients who have Graves' disease. Because LATS can cross the placenta, LATS levels should be obtained from such patients, and the pediatrician should be alerted to possible neonatal thyrotoxicosis if LATS is present.

**208. The answer is B (1, 3).** *(Pritchard, ed 16. pp 767-768.)* Toxoplasmosis, a protozoal infection caused by *Toxoplasma gondii*, can result from ingestion of raw or undercooked meat infected by the organism or from contact with infected cat feces. Its incidence in pregnant women is estimated to be 1 in every 150 to 700 pregnancies. Infection early in pregnancy may cause abortion; later in pregnancy, however, the fetus may become infected. A small number of infected infants develop involvement of the central nervous system or the eye; most infants who have the disease, however, escape serious clinical problems.

**209. The answer is D (4).** *(Burrow, p 820.)* Phenylketonuria is a rare disorder that results from a deficiency in the liver enzyme that catalyzes the conversion of phenylalanine to tyrosine. The resultant high levels of phenylalanine can cause damage to the developing brain. Thus, the chance that a women who has phenylketonuria will have a retarded child is almost 100 percent if her blood levels of phenylalanine are not kept within normal limits. These retarded offspring rarely have the disease themselves. The institution of a low-phenylalanine diet **before** conception may prevent the development of retardation, if the diet is continued throughout pregnancy, but the evidence of this is uncertain. A low-phenylalanine diet begun **after** conception, however, seems to be of no value in preventing retardation. Because of the high risk of severe mental retardation in affected offspring, interruption of pregnancy has been recommended for women who have phenylketonuria and either have never been placed on low-phenylalanine diets or were started on their diets after becoming pregnant.

**210. The answer is E (all).** *(Burrow, pp 182-184.)* Maternal diabetes, especially of the milder classes, is associated with macrosomia in the fetus. Glucose crosses the placenta freely by facilitated diffusion, but insulin does not. The fetus, in response to the chronic glucose load, secretes increased quantities of insulin. Insulin acts as a growth hormone in the fetus, and the fetus becomes macrosomic. At delivery, the fetus is removed from the relatively glucose-rich maternal environment but continues to secrete increased amounts of insulin. Thus, the fetus may become hypoglycemic in the early hours of life unless early feeding, sometimes even intravenous glucose, is begun. Hypocalcemia may occur in as many as one fourth of infants of diabetic mothers, possibly as a result of fetal parathyroid suppression stemming from maternal hypercalcemia. Lastly, fetal lung maturity, as measured by the lecithin-to-sphingomyelin ratio, may be delayed, especially in the infants of mothers who have mild diabetes.

**211. The answer is A (1, 2, 3).** *(Burrow, pp 173, 181-186.)* Sophisticated management of high-risk diabetic individuals has reduced the incidence of diabetic ketoacidosis. When it occurs in pregnant women, however, it is associated with an extremely high fetal mortality rate. In addition, ketonuria in the absence of acidosis (i.e., starvation ketosis) has been correlated with decreased intelligence quotients in the offspring. Perinatal mortality has been correlated to hyperglycemia even in the absence of ketoacidosis, and this finding is the cornerstone of current recommendations urging strict control of diabetes during pregnancy. A correlation between maternal hypoglycemia and fetal morbidity or mortality has not been shown; in fact, rather severe episodes of hypoglycemia have been reported to have no effect on the outcome of pregnancy.

**212. The answer is B (1, 3).** *(Pritchard, ed 16. pp 949-952.)* Although all infants beyond 42 weeks gestation are considered postmature, the postmaturity syndrome does not affect all these infants. The syndrome itself consists of wasted subcutaneous tissues, peeling skin, long nails, diminished amniotic fluid, and meconium staining of amniotic fluid and baby. Prior to birth, ultrasound examination can detect a decreased amniotic fluid volume, and amniocentesis can be used to determine the presence or absence of meconium. The presence of postmaturity syndrome correlates with an increase in the stillbirth rate and an increase in neonatal complications, the most common of which are meconium aspiration and hypoglycemia. The incidence of cord entanglement also is increased, probably due to diminished amniotic fluid volumes. When gestation is prolonged beyond the forty-second week of pregnancy and meconium or oligohydramnios is present, prompt delivery should be performed.

**213. The answer is E (all).** *(Burrow, pp 416-433, 479.)* A mild group B coxsackievirus infection of the mother during the antepartum period may give rise to a virulent infection in the newborn, sometimes resulting in a fatal encephalomyocarditis. A maternal rubella infection may cause neonatal hepatosplenomegaly, petechial rash, and jaundice; in addition, viral shedding may last for months or years. Herpes zoster, the causative agent of varicella (chickenpox), is an especially dangerous organism for the newborn. Varicella is rare in pregnancy, but if it occurs shortly before delivery, the viremia may spread to the fetus before protective maternal antibodies have had a chance to form. Congenital varicella can be fatal to the newborn; the increasing availability of zoster immunoglobulin, however, may allow clinicians to attack the infection before significant fetal viremia has developed. Herpesvirus can be acquired by the fetus as it passes down the genital tract and can cause a severe, often fatal herpes infection in the newborn.

**214. The answer is C (2, 4).** *(Pritchard, ed 16. pp 185-187.)* Immunoglobulin G (IgG) easily crosses the placenta and thus is found in approximately equal amounts in maternal and fetal blood. Immunoglobulin M (IgM), on the other hand, is a large molecule and does not cross the placenta. Thus maternal levels of IgM are higher than fetal levels, unless an intrauterine infection causes the fetus to manufacture IgM. The gamma chains in hemoglobin (Hb) are what distinguish fetal hemoglobin from adult hemoglobin. Fetal hemoglobin (Hb F) contains two alpha and two gamma chains. Hb A, found in most adults, contains two alpha and two beta chains. One would therefore expect to find more gamma chains in the fetal blood than in maternal blood. Finally, cord-blood fibrinogen levels are normally quite low; maternal fibrinogen levels, on the other hand, are about 50 percent higher than levels in nonpregnant women.

**215. The answer is D (4).** *(Burrow, pp 919-923.)* The lecithin-to-sphingomyelin (L/S) ratio, measured from amniotic-fluid samples, is a barometer of pulmonic maturity. If the L/S ratio is above whatever value denotes maturity in a particular laboratory, respiratory distress syndrome will probably not be present in the newborn. Lecithin seems to be involved in surfactant activity, and its secretion from the lungs into the amniotic fluid yields information about surfactant production in the fetal lungs. Amniotic-fluid creatinine values have been used to document fetal maturity; but because they also can reflect the muscle mass of a fetus, they are not as valid as the L/S ratio. The L/S ratio may reach maturity levels earlier in stressful situations, as in toxemia of pregnancy. Delay in pulmonic maturation occurs in association with mild diabetes but not with erythroblastosis fetalis.

216. **The answer is C (2, 4).** *(Aladjem, ed 2. pp 56-62.)* Fetal heart rate has been shown to drop almost immediately when the umbilical circulation has been obstructed in experimental situations. This response is a reflex action that is caused by the sudden rise in central venous pressure and that disappears if the vagi are severed. A more prolonged obstruction of the umbilical circulation can cause a delayed fall in the fetal heart rate secondary to progressive asphyxia.

217. **The answer is B (1, 3).** *(Benirschke, NY State J Med 61:4499, 1961.)* The twin-twin transfusion syndrome is a result of vascular anastomoses between the arterial circulation of one twin and the venous circulation of the other. Because a monochorionic placenta must be present, dizygotic twins are not affected by the twin-twin transfusion syndrome, even if their placentas are fused.

218. **The answer is D (4).** *(Pritchard, ed 16. pp 639-640.)* Monozygotic twins are formed from the splitting of a single fertilized ovum and occur in approximately 1 birth in 250. Dizygotic twins, which are more common, result from multiple ovulations during the same menstrual cycle. The incidence of monozygotic twinning seems to be relatively constant despite differences in race, heredity, age, and hormonal therapy. Dizygotic twinning, on the other hand, is influenced by all of these factors; it occurs more commonly in blacks than in whites, seems to run (by the maternal-hereditary line) in families, and is more common with increasing age and parity. The use of clomiphene for ovulation induction is associated with multiple ovulation and an approximately 7-percent incidence of multiple gestation (as opposed to approximately 1.0 to 1.4 percent in the normal population). The use of gonadotropins to stimulate ovulation is associated with an even higher incidence of multiple gestations, with some series reporting as high as 40 percent.

219-222. **The answers are: 219-A, 220-C, 221-A, 222-B.** *(Pritchard, ed 16. pp 180-182, 203-206.)* Oxygen travels from mother to fetus, and carbon dioxide from fetus to mother, by **simple diffusion** across the placenta. Carbon dioxide travels more rapidly than oxygen, probably because fetal and maternal blood have different affinities for these two substances. Iron is **actively transported** (i.e., in an energy-requiring process) from mother to fetus; as a result, the mother may become markedly iron-depleted during pregnancy, while the fetus does well. Glucose crosses to the fetus by **facilitated diffusion**, which means that its transfer across the placenta is more rapid than could be accounted for by simple diffusion alone. The fetus acts as a "glucose sink," continuously obtaining glucose at the expense of the mother. This fact may help to explain the lower-than-normal levels of maternal fasting blood glucose found during pregnancy. **Pinocytosis** describes the process by which liquid is imbibed by cells as a result of invagination of the cell membrane.

# Pregnancy, Labor, Delivery, and Puerperium

**DIRECTIONS**: Each question below contains five suggested answers. Choose the **one best** response to each question.

223. A pregnant woman is seen 18 days after she has been exposed to rubella. Her hemagglutination inhibition titer is 1:8. Her physician should

(A) administer rubella vaccine
(B) recommend an abortion
(C) repeat the titer 2 days later
(D) repeat the titer 10 to 14 days later
(E) obtain weekly titers for the next 4 weeks

224. A pregnant woman is discovered to be an asymptomatic carrier of *Neisseria gonorrhoeae*. A year ago, she was treated with penicillin for a gonococcal infection and developed a severe allergic reaction. Treatment of choice at this time would be

(A) tetracycline
(B) ampicillin
(C) erythromycin
(D) spectinomycin
(E) chloramphenicol

225. A multiparous woman is one who has completed

(A) two or more pregnancies, regardless of the length of gestation
(B) two or more pregnancies reaching the stage of viability
(C) two or more pregnancies resulting in delivery
(D) two or more pregnancies resulting in delivery of liveborn infants
(E) a single pregnancy resulting in a multiple birth

226. The oxytocin challenge test is considered negative if

(A) at least three uterine contractions occur in a 10-minute interval and late deceleration of fetal heart rate is absent
(B) at least three uterine contractions occur in a 10-minute interval and late deceleration is inconsistent
(C) less than three uterine contractions occur in a 10-minute interval, regardless of whether late deceleration occurs
(D) the uterus contracts at least once every 2 minutes, regardless of whether late deceleration occurs
(E) no uterine contractions are noted

227. A 25-year-old woman, gravida 1, para 0, who has a history of infertility, comes to your office at 20 weeks gestation. Her uterus is enlarged (24 weeks). She was treated in the past with a fertility drug, the name of which she does not know. You obtain an ultrasonogram, which is shown below. The most likely diagnosis is

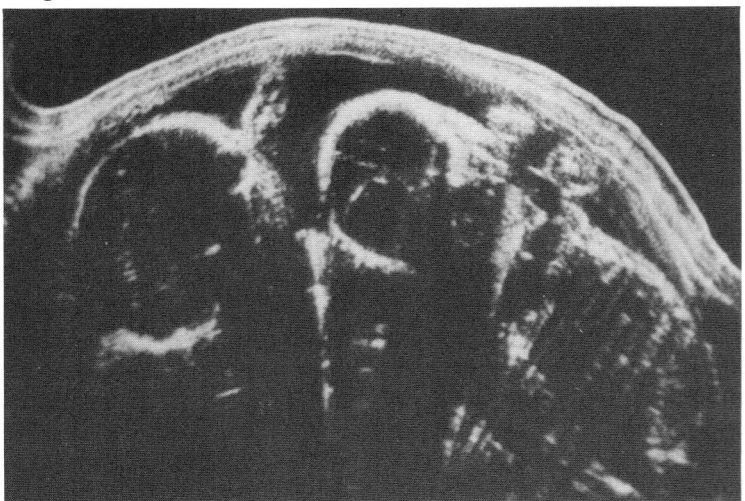

(A) hydatidiform mole
(B) placenta previa
(C) anencephalic fetus
(D) twins
(E) normal single-fetus pregnancy

228. Which of the following statements about frank breech presentation is true?

(A) It is less common than complete breech presentation
(B) It is less common than incomplete breech presentation
(C) The lower extremities are flexed at the hips but extended at the knees
(D) The hips and one or both knees are flexed
(E) The feet often can be palpated beside the buttocks

229. The major reason that birth-control pills are contraindicated for lactating mothers is their association with

(A) fibrocystic disease of the breast
(B) carcinoma of the breast
(C) thromboembolism in the newborn
(D) subsequent onset of juvenile diabetes
(E) jaundice in the newborn

230. The x-ray shown below, which was taken in the plane of the pelvic inlet, demonstrates which of the following types of pelvic morphology?

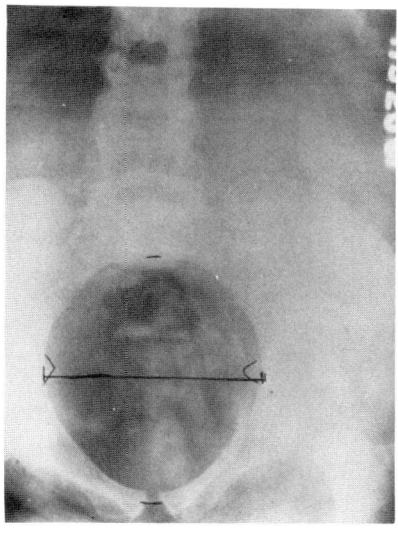

(A) Anthropoid
(B) Android
(C) Gynecoid
(D) Platypelloid
(E) Trianguloid

231. The cardinal movements of labor occur in which of the following sequences?

(A) Flexion, descent, internal rotation, external rotation, and extension
(B) Flexion, descent, external rotation, internal rotation, and extension
(C) Flexion, internal rotation, descent, extension, and external rotation
(D) Descent, flexion, internal rotation, extension, and external rotation
(E) Descent, flexion, external rotation, extension, and internal rotation

232. Which of the following statements about the third stage of labor is true?

(A) It is defined as the hour immediately following the delivery of the placenta
(B) The earliest clinical sign is that the uterus has become globular and firm
(C) Forced placental expression before placental separation often is beneficial
(D) There is less blood loss than normal with the Duncan mechanism of placental expression
(E) There is less blood loss than normal with Schultze's mechanism of placental expression

## Questions 233-235

The sketch shown below details the major landmarks of the fetal skull as it presents in the maternal pelvis. The perspective is that of the obstetrician facing the perineum.

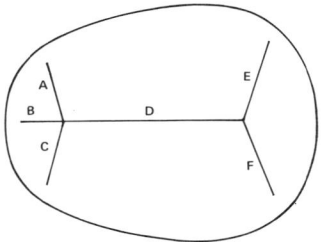

233. The position of the fetal vertex is

(A) left occiput anterior
(B) left sacrum transverse
(C) left occiput transverse
(D) right occiput transverse
(E) mentum posterior

234. The lambdoid sutures are

(A) **A** and **C**
(B) **A, C,** and **D**
(C) **B** and **D**
(D) **E** and **F**
(E) none of the above

235. The intersection of **D, E,** and **F** forms the

(A) caput succedaneum
(B) parietal prominence
(C) biparietal plane
(D) anterior fontanelle
(E) posterior fontanelle

236. Which line on the echogram shown below represents the biparietal diameter of the fetal skull?

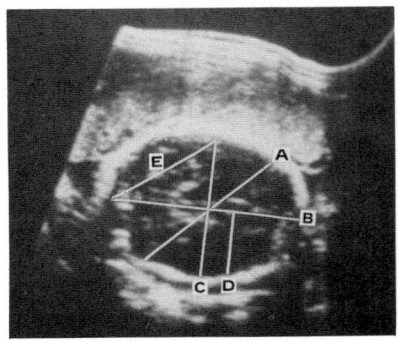

(A) Line A
(B) Line B
(C) Line C
(D) Line D
(E) Line E

**DIRECTIONS**: Each question below contains four suggested answers of which **one** or **more** is correct. Choose the answer:

|   |    |                |             |
|---|----|----------------|-------------|
| A | if | 1, 2, and 3    | are correct |
| B | if | 1 and 3        | are correct |
| C | if | 2 and 4        | are correct |
| D | if | 4              | is correct  |
| E | if | 1, 2, 3, and 4 | are correct |

237. Appropriate measures in the treatment of women who have edema of pregnancy include

(1) salt restriction
(2) weight control
(3) diuretics
(4) bed rest

238. The use of which of the following antibiotics is contraindicated during pregnancy?

(1) Tetracycline
(2) Penicillin
(3) Chloramphenicol
(4) Ampicillin

239. A young primigravid woman is found to have asymptomatic *Escherichia coli* bacteriuria at her first prenatal visit. True statements about this woman include which of the following?

(1) She is at risk for delivering prematurely
(2) She is at risk for developing pyelonephritis
(3) She is at risk for developing pregnancy-induced hypertension
(4) She should be treated with oral antibiotics

240. Positive signs of pregnancy include which of the following?

(1) Ultrasonographic visualization of the fetal head
(2) Detection of the funic souffle
(3) Perception of fetal movements by an experienced examiner
(4) Positive urine test for chorionic gonadotropin

241. True statements about the oxytocin challenge test include which of the following?

(1) It determines the inducibility of the uterus
(2) Its effects are measured by internal monitors
(3) It is considered positive if the uterus contracts once every 2 minutes
(4) It can serve as a fetal stress test

242. Prerequisites for application of forceps include

(1) complete dilation of the cervix
(2) engagement of the fetal head
(3) ruptured membranes
(4) vertex or face presentation

## SUMMARY OF DIRECTIONS

| A | B | C | D | E |
|---|---|---|---|---|
| 1, 2, 3 only | 1, 3 only | 2, 4 only | 4 only | All are correct |

243. In a lower uterine segment cesarean section, the advantages of a transverse incision as compared with a vertical incision include

(1) less blood loss
(2) less likelihood of extending into the broad ligaments
(3) less likelihood of extending into the cervix and vagina
(4) more room for extraction of the fetus

244. Obstetrical analgesia and anesthesia can be described by which of the following statements?

(1) The most common cause of death due to anesthesia is pneumonitis from aspirated gastric material and juices
(2) Intravenous thiopental and other barbiturates are relatively ineffective in producing analgesia and can cause depression in the newborn infant
(3) Antacids given before general anesthesia can diminish the risk of serious pulmonary injury
(4) Naloxone, a narcotic antagonist, is effective only against respiratory depression induced by opioid narcotics

245. Which of the following circumstances should alert an obstetrician to an increased likelihood of postpartum hemorrhage?

(1) Prolonged labor
(2) Rapid labor
(3) Oxytocin stimulation of labor
(4) Twin pregnancy

246. Signs of placental separation include which of the following?

(1) Lengthening of the umbilical cord
(2) Change in the shape of the uterus from globular to discoid
(3) Sudden gush of blood
(4) Strong uterine contractions

247. True statements about $Rh_o(D)$ immune globulin (RhoGAM) include which of the following?

(1) Administration is therapeutically unsuccessful in approximately 1.5 percent of cases
(2) It should never be administered during pregnancy
(3) It usually is given in a dose of 300 $\mu$g within 72 hours of delivery of an Rh-positive infant to an unsensitized Rh-negative woman
(4) It can prevent ABO (blood group) incompatibility

DIRECTIONS: The group of questions below consists of lettered choices followed by several numbered items. For each numbered item select the one lettered choice with which it is most closely associated. Each lettered choice may be used once, more than once, or not at all.

Questions 248-252

The safety of immunization during pregnancy is a matter of concern and controversy that has prompted the American College of Obstetricians and Gynecologists to offer specific recommendations for the use of immunization therapy for pregnant women. For each disease vaccine listed below, select the recommendation with which it is most likely to be associated.

(A) Recommended if the underlying disease is serious
(B) Recommended after exposure or before travel to endemic areas
(C) Not routinely recommended but mandatory during an epidemic
(D) Contraindicated unless exposure to the disease is unavoidable
(E) Contraindicated

248. Poliomyelitis
249. Mumps
250. Influenza
251. Rubella
252. Hepatitis A

# Pregnancy, Labor, Delivery, and Puerperium

# Answers

**223. The answer is D.** *(Burrow, pp 420, 423.)* A titer of 1:8 obtained by a hemagglutination inhibition test may or may not indicate prior exposure to rubella virus. This titer in an exposed patient could represent a false positive result caused by the presence of nonspecific hemagglutinin inhibitors, which can be found in all human sera. On the other hand, a patient who has a titer of 1:8 18 days after exposure to rubella could be susceptible and harboring an inapparent infection that has just begun to stimulate manufacture of antibody. If a titer repeated 10 to 14 days later is the same as the first one, the patient is assumed to be immune. If, on the other hand, the repeat titer is 1:32 or greater, the initial titer most likely represented early antibody response to an inapparent infection. Rubella vaccination is contraindicated in pregnant woman.

**224. The answer is C.** *(Monif, p 8.)* Erythromycin is the treatment of choice for pregnant women who have an asymptomatic *Neisseria gonorrhoeae* infection and who are allergic to penicillin. Although tetracycline also is an effective alternative to penicillin, its use is contraindicated in pregnancy. Spectinomycin is another drug effective in treating asymptomatic gonorrhea, but erythromycin is preferred in pregnant women because of uncertain effects of spectinomycin on the fetus. Administration of chloramphenicol is not recommended to treat women, pregnant or not, who have cervical gonorrhea, and the use of ampicillin is contraindicated for penicillin-allergic patients.

**225. The answer is B.** *(Pritchard, ed 16. p 304.)* Parity is determined by the number of pregnancies that have reached viability (i.e., beyond the stage of abortion) and not by the number of deliveries. Parity is not increased by a multiple birth or decreased by a stillbirth. A primipara is a woman who has been delivered of a viable fetus once; a multipara has completed at least two viable pregnancies.

Pregnancy, Delivery, and Puerperium

**226. The answer is A.** *(Pritchard, ed 16. pp 349-352.)* The oxytocin challenge test is negative if the uterus contracts at least three times in a 10-minute interval, if each contraction lasts 40 seconds or longer, and if the contractions are not accompanied by a late deceleration of the fetal heart rate. Test results should be considered suspicious if late deceleration is uneven and unsustained in spite of continuing uterine contractions. In the presence of hyperstimulation of the uterus, judged either by the contraction frequency (more than one every 2 minutes) or length (longer than 90 seconds), late deceleration of the fetal heart rate may not signify uteroplacental disease.

**227. The answer is D.** *(Pritchard, ed 16. pp 648-651.)* The ultrasonogram presented in the question clearly shows twins. The diagnosis can be made by noting the two heads (the circular densities). A hydatidiform mole would show no evidence of fetal parts or cranium. The presence of a spherical cranium rules out anencephaly. Because the placenta is anterior and superior, placenta previa is not present. Ultrasound has been very helpful in the diagnosis, early in gestation, of twins.

**228. The answer is C.** *(Pritchard, ed 16. pp 797-807.)* The position of the lower extremities relative to the buttocks helps determine the descriptive presentation of the breech. Frank breech presentation is characterized by flexion of the lower extremities at the hips and extension at the knees. With a complete breech presentation, the hips and one or both knees are flexed; often, feet can be felt beside the buttocks. In incomplete breech presentation, the hips are not flexed and at least one foot or knee lies below the breech. Radiographic diagnosis of frank breech presentation is more common than either complete or incomplete breech.

**229. The answer is E.** *(Wynn, ed 2. p 235.)* The synthetic sex steroids used in oral contraceptives may easily cross to the newborn in breast milk and cause jaundice in the newborn as well as other, as-yet-unrecognized effects. Other undesirable effects include suppression of lactation and increased risk of maternal thromboembolism in the early postpartum period. The pill has been associated with a decreased incidence of fibrocystic disease of the breast, but no association with breast cancer has been shown. Further, there is no known relationship to subsequent diabetes or an increase in thromboembolism in the newborn.

**230. The answer is A.** *(Pritchard, ed 16. pp 286-288.)* The anteroposterior diameter of the inlet of the anthropoid pelvis shown in the x-ray is greater than the transverse diameter. The anterior segment of an anthropoid pelvis is narrow, the ischial spines often are prominent, and the side walls may be somewhat convergent. In one American study, the anthropoid pelvis was found to be nearly twice as common (40 percent to 23 percent) in nonwhite women as in white women. This type of pelvis is far more likely than a gynecoid pelvis to be a source of dystocia.

**231. The answer is D.** *(Pritchard, ed 16. pp 396-402.)* Although the cardinal movements of labor do not necessarily follow one after another, they may be sequenced to aid in understanding labor's underlying mechanisms. The head generally enters the pelvis as an occiput transverse presentation, due to the usual configuration of the inlet. As it **descends** into the pelvis, **flexion** occurs. As the head passes the midplane, the musculature of the pelvic floor causes **internal rotation**, or movement from occiput transverse to occiput anterior (or posterior). As the occiput passes under the symphysis and comes in contact with the perineum, **extension** occurs, allowing delivery of the head. As the shoulders pass into the pelvis, they align in the anteroposterior plane, causing the head to go back to the occiput transverse position, a process called **external rotation**.

**232. The answer is B.** *(Pritchard, ed 16. pp 389-390.)* The third stage of labor is the period between delivery of the infant and separation of the placenta. The characteristic signs of placental separation usually occur within 5 minutes of delivery; in order of appearance, these signs include firming of a globular uterus, a gush of blood, uterine ascent in the abdomen, and lengthening of the umbilical cord. Forced expression of the placenta before it has separated can be dangerous, because it can cause inversion of the uterus. Schultze's mechanism and the Duncan mechanism refer to variations of placental expulsion; neither is associated with decreased blood loss.

**233-235. The answers are: 233-C, 234-D, 235-E.** *(Pritchard, ed 16. pp 176, 293-297.)* A good knowledge of the major landmarks of the fetal skull is essential for anyone performing deliveries. The position of the fetal vertex in the accompanying sketch is left occiput transverse. The lambdoid sutures (**E** and **F**) meet the sagittal suture (**D**) to form the posterior fontanelle. The occiput is just posterior to the posterior fontanelle. The posterior, or Y-shaped, fontanelle is the reference point for vertex presentations. The side of the maternal pelvis to which it is closest defines the position. The head is oriented in a transverse (or horizontal) manner, with the occiput nearest the maternal left side; thus, this is left occiput transverse. The anterior, or diamond-shaped, fontanelle is made up of the intersection of the sagittal, frontal (**B**), and the two coronal (**A** and **C**) sutures. Extreme molding of the fetal head may make identification of these landmarks very difficult. Other clues to the position of the head include abdominal palpation of the back and small parts and, more important, palpation of an ear. If an ear can be felt and the relationship between the locations of the pinna and the auditory canal can be ascertained, the position of the vertex can be deduced.

Pregnancy, Delivery, and Puerperium 107

**236. The answer is C.** *(Pritchard, ed 16. p 345.)* The biparietal diameter is figured from the inner table of one area of the fetal skull (one echo) to the outer table of the other. In the echogram shown, the falx is easily seen in the midline. Therefore, line C represents the true biparietal diameter. Line A represents a diagonal from one table of the skull to another. Line B measures the longitudinal length of the skull. Line D represents the distance between the falx and the outer table of the fetal skull, and line E is a chord describing a portion of the circumference. The measurement of the biparietal diameter is essential to modern-day obstetricians because it can establish intrauterine gestational age.

**237. The answer is C (2, 4).** *(Burrow, pp 929-930. Romney, p 687.)* Edema is present to a greater or lesser degree in all pregnant women but most frequently among women who gain an excessive amount of weight. Edema of pregnancy has traditionally been treated with salt restriction and diuretics; however, it is now clear that sodium and water retention are normal processes during pregnancy. More water than sodium is retained, so unnecessary salt restriction and diuretics may cause intravascular depletion. Diuretics also may cause sodium and potassium depletion in the mother. Thiazide diuretics have been implicated in hemorrhagic pancreatitis and deterioration of glucose tolerance in the mother and in thrombocytopenia in the newborn. The best treatment for edema of pregnancy is bed rest in the lateral recumbent position, which should improve renal perfusion, and weight control if obesity is the major problem.

**238. The answer is B (1, 3).** *(Monif, pp 19-26.)* Tetracycline may cause fetal dental anomalies and inhibition of bone growth if administered during the second trimester, and it is a potential teratogen to first-trimester fetuses. Tetracycline administration also can cause severe hepatic decompensation in the mother, especially during the third trimester. Chloramphenicol may cause the "gray baby" syndrome (symptoms of which include vomiting, impaired respiration, hypothermia, and, finally, cardiovascular collapse) in neonates who have received large doses of the drug. No notable adverse effects have been associated with the use of penicillin or ampicillin.

**239. The answer is C (2, 4).** *(Monif, pp 322-323.)* Women who have asymptomatic bacteriuria have a 20- to 30-percent chance of developing pyelonephritis and therefore should be treated with oral antibiotics. Most cases of pyelonephritis of pregnancy could be prevented by treating asymptomatic bacteriuria. The relationship between asymptomatic bacteriuria and other complications, such as premature labor and toxemia of pregnancy, has been suggested but not clearly established.

240. The answer is A (1, 2, 3). *(Pritchard, ed 16. pp 261-264.)* Ultrasonographic visualization of the fetal head, which is generally possible by 14 weeks menstrual age, is an unmistakable sign of pregnancy. Earlier identification of the gestational "ring," which may occur at 6 to 8 weeks, does not necessarily imply a true pregnancy, because a blighted ovum could present the same appearance. Detection of the funic (umbilical-cord) souffle is a positive sign of pregnancy, because cord pulsations are synchronous with the fetal heart beat. The uterine souffle, on the other hand, is synchronous with the maternal heart rate and does not necessarily imply pregnancy. Perception of fetal movements by an experienced examiner also is diagnostic of pregnancy. A positive urinary (or serum) chorionic gonadotropin (or beta subunit) level is not diagnostic of pregnancy; hydatidiform mole and other tumors may produce this hormone.

241. The answer is D (4). *(Pritchard, ed 16. pp 349-352.)* The oxytocin challenge test assesses the ability of the fetoplacental unit to withstand the stress of labor. After external monitors have measured the baseline activity of the uterus and fetal heart for 10 minutes, intravenous oxytocin is infused at a rate of 0.5 milliunits per minute. The rate is doubled every 15 to 20 minutes until three contractions, each of which last for 40 to 60 seconds, occur every 10 minutes. The test is considered positive if fetal heart rate consistently decelerates once uterine contractions have begun.

242. The answer is E (all). *(Pritchard, ed 16. pp 1042-1044.)* Prerequisites for application of forceps include engagement of the fetal head, full cervical dilation, ruptured membranes, knowledge of the position of the presenting part, fetal presentation as either vertex or face (mentum anterior), and sufficient pelvic dimensions allowing a vaginal delivery. If the forceps are applied prior to engagement, trauma to maternal organs and injury to the fetus are possible. Delivery of the unengaged head should be by cesarean section. If the cervix is not fully dilated, severe cervical lacerations, including intra-abdominal trauma, may result. If the membranes are unruptured, the forceps can slip around the head. If the position of the presenting part is not established, injury to the fetus can result.

243. The answer is B (1, 3). *(Pritchard, ed 16. p 1085.)* In a lower uterine segment cesarean section, a transverse incision results in less blood loss, because it goes through the thinned-out lower uterine segment and does not involve much of the myometrium, site of the large blood vessels. (However, if the placenta is implanted over the anterior lower uterine segment, blood loss can be significant.) The transverse incision also is less likely to extend into the cervix and vagina, because its direction of extension is usually horizontal. A transverse incision is more likely than a vertical incision to extend into the broad ligaments. If this happens, catastrophic hemorrhage can result. A vertical incision actually allows

more room for extraction of the fetus, because it can extend upward toward the fundus. Many obstetricians prefer the vertical incision in situations where extra room is needed, as for example, in a breech presentation.

**244. The answer is E (all).** *(Pritchard, ed 16. pp 435-442.)* In obstetrics, death from anesthesia most commonly results from pneumonitis caused by the inhalation of gastric acid. Administration of antacids before general anesthesia can lessen gastric acidity and therefore reduce the risk of serious pulmonary injury. The use of intravenous thiopental or other barbiturates, which are rather ineffective analgesics, can cause significant respiratory depression in the newborn. Narcotic antagonists, such as naloxone, levallorphan, and nalorphine, are effective only in reducing respiratory depression caused by opioid narcotics.

**245. The answer is E (all).** *(Pritchard, ed 16. pp 877-879.)* Prolonged or rapid labor, oxytocin stimulation of labor, and twin pregnancy all predispose to uterine atony and, thus, to postpartum hemorrhage. A uterus that has required oxytocin in order to provide adequate labor is likely to need large amounts of oxytocin afterwards in order to stay contracted. A uterus that has stretched to accommodate twin gestations is likely to be atonic after it is emptied. No explanation is given for the clinical finding that a uterus that has been hypertonic and yielded a rapid labor is predisposed to atony.

**246. The answer is B (1, 3).** *(Pritchard, ed 16. p 423.)* The usual signs of placental separation include lengthening of the umbilical cord, a sudden gush of blood, a change in the shape of the uterus from discoid to globular, and the rising up of the uterus in the abdomen. Attempts to deliver the placenta before separation may cause serious problems, such as inversion of the uterus or avulsion of the cord. One useful way to avoid inverting the uterus is to wait until the placenta has separated and is in the lower uterine segment and then to perform the Brandt (or Brandt-Andrews) maneuver, pressing upward on the fundus from the suprapubic region while gently exerting cord traction.

**247. The answer is B (1, 3).** *(Scott, Contemporary Obstet Gynecol 8:27, 1976.)* $Rh_o(D)$ immune globulin (RhoGAM) is a concentrated sterile solution of human immunoglobulin G that contains anti-$Rh_o(D)$; it can prevent the formation of active $Rh_o(D)$ antibody in women, thereby impeding the development of Rh hemolytic disease of the newborn in subsequent deliveries. $Rh_o(D)$ immune globulin is usually given in an intramuscular dose of 300 µg within 72 hours of delivery. The failure rate, which is reported to be 1 to 2 percent, is attributed either to the development of sensitization in a subsequent pregnancy or to an unrecognized sensitization that already exists when the drug is administered. $Rh_o(D)$ immune globulin is of no benefit in ABO (blood group) incompatibility.

248-252. The answers are: 248-C, 249-E, 250-A, 251-E, 252-B. *(Pritchard, ed 16. p 321.)* The recommendations concerning immunization during pregnancy offered by the American College of Obstetricians and Gynecologists are as follows:

(1) Administration of influenza vaccine is recommended if the underlying disease is serious.

(2) Typhoid immunization is recommended when traveling to an endemic region.

(3) Hepatitis A immunization is recommended after exposure or before travel to developing countries.

(4) Cholera immunization should be given only to meet travel requirements.

(5) Tetanus-diphtheria immunization should be given if a primary series has never been administered or if 10 years have elapsed without receiving a booster.

(6) Immunization for poliomyelitis is mandatory during an epidemic but otherwise not recommended.

(7) Smallpox immunization is unnecessary since the disease has been eradicated.

(8) Immunization for yellow fever is recommended before travel to a high-risk area.

(9) Mumps and rubella immunization is contraindicated.

(10) Administration of rabies vaccine is unaffected by pregnancy.

# ABNORMALITIES OF PREGNANCY

# Spontaneous Abortion, Ectopic Pregnancies, and Trophoblastic Disease

**DIRECTIONS**: Each question below contains five suggested answers. Choose the one best response to each question.

253. The chromosomal abnormality most often detected in first trimester abortuses is

(A) Turner's syndrome
(B) polyploidy
(C) autosomal monosomy
(D) autosomal trisomy
(E) unbalanced translocation

254. All of the following statements about ectopic tubal pregnancy are true EXCEPT that

(A) abdominal pain and bleeding are the most consistent findings
(B) the initial pain usually is intermittent and crampy
(C) the involved tube usually is grossly normal
(D) amenorrhea is present in more than 90 percent of affected women
(E) most abdominal pregnancies are "aborted" tubal pregnancies

255. Heart tones could not be detected from a fetus at 22 weeks of gestation. Amniography was ordered, and the x-ray shown below was obtained. The diagnosis is

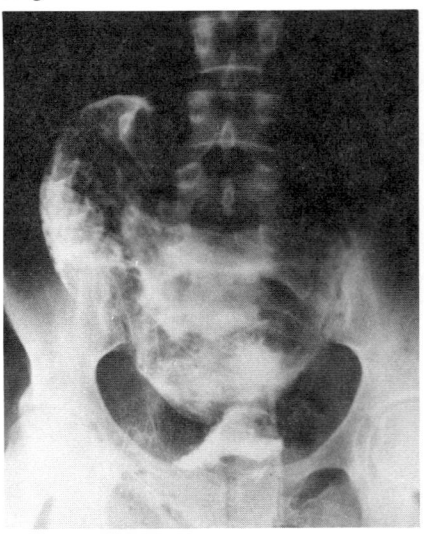

(A) hydatidiform mole
(B) normal intrauterine pregnancy
(C) ovarian cystadenocarcinoma
(D) abdominal pregnancy
(E) pseudocyesis

256. A 19-year-old woman comes to the emergency room and reports that she had passed out at work earlier in the day. She has mild vaginal bleeding, and her abdomen is diffusely tender and distended. In addition, she complains of shoulder and abdominal pain. Temperature is 36.4°C (97.6°F); pulse rate, 120 per minute; and blood pressure, 96/50 mm Hg. To confirm the diagnosis suggested by the available clinical data, which of the following diagnostic procedures would best be utilized?

(A) A pregnancy test
(B) Posterior colpotomy
(C) Dilatation and curettage
(D) Culdocentesis
(E) Laparoscopy

257. A 32-year-old woman, gravida 3, para 3, presents with abdominal pain. Her last menstrual period was 6 weeks ago, and a pregnancy test is positive. The specimen shown below is obtained at laparotomy. The most likely diagnosis is

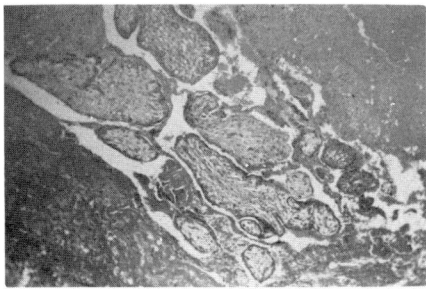

(A) incomplete abortion
(B) missed abortion
(C) hydatidiform mole
(D) tubal ectopic pregnancy
(E) none of the above

258. All of the following statements about abdominal pregnancy are true EXCEPT that

(A) secondary implantations are more common than primary
(B) symptoms include abdominal discomfort and fetal movements in the abdomen
(C) it can be diagnosed by failure of oxytocin induction of labor
(D) ultrasound is a safe and effective means of diagnosis
(E) the placenta should be removed at the time of delivery to prevent eventual uncontrolled hemorrhage

259. All of the following statements concerning ectopic pregnancy are true EXCEPT that

(A) it occurs more commonly among black women than white women
(B) the fallopian tube is the most common site of implantation
(C) if a woman has had a tubal pregnancy or undergone tubal plastic surgery, the chance of having a future ectopic pregnancy is 10 to 20 times greater than in the general population
(D) one of the most important etiological factors is pelvic inflammatory disease
(E) its incidence in women who have pelvic inflammatory disease is decreased by the use of conventional antibiotic therapy

**Questions 260-262**

A 19-year-old primigravid woman is expecting her first child; she is 12 weeks pregnant by dates. She has vaginal bleeding and an enlarged-for-dates uterus. In addition, no fetal heart sounds are heard. A sample of tissue that she has passed vaginally is shown below.

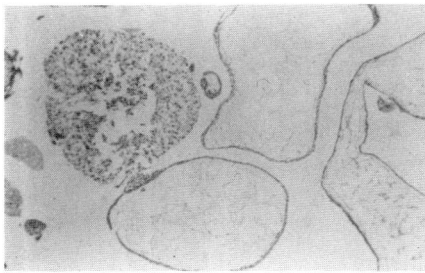

260. The most likely diagnosis of this woman's condition is

(A) sarcoma botryoides
(B) tuberculous endometritis
(C) adenocarcinoma of the uterus
(D) hydatidiform mole
(E) normal pregnancy

261. The safest and most reliable method for early diagnosis of this woman's condition is

(A) amniography
(B) ultrasonography
(C) abdominal roentgenogram
(D) pelvic arteriography
(E) human chorionic gonadotropin (HCG) titer

262. After uterine evacuation, management of the woman described above who has no clinical or radiographic evidence of metastatic disease should include

(A) weekly HCG titers
(B) hysterectomy
(C) single-agent chemotherapy
(D) combination chemotherapy
(E) radiation therapy

263. The presence of adnexal masses in a woman who has a hydatidiform mole is an indication for

(A) hormone therapy
(B) radiation therapy
(C) emergency surgical intervention
(D) eventual surgical intervention
(E) none of the above

**DIRECTIONS**: Each question below contains four suggested answers of which **one** or **more** is correct. Choose the answer:

| A | if | 1, 2, and 3 | are correct |
|---|----|-------------|-------------|
| B | if | 1 and 3 | are correct |
| C | if | 2 and 4 | are correct |
| D | if | 4 | is correct |
| E | if | 1, 2, 3, and 4 | are correct |

264. Disorders referred to as gestational trophoblastic disease include

(1) hydatidiform mole
(2) chorioadenoma destruens
(3) choriocarcinoma
(4) ovarian choriocarcinoma

265. Determination of the presence of a growing tumor in a patient who has gestational trophoblastic disease could be established by

(1) serial chest x-rays
(2) evaluation of menstrual function
(3) presence of lactation
(4) serial HCG titers

266. The histological classification of gestational trophoblastic disease can be characterized by which of the following statements?

(1) It is a reliable indicator of prognosis
(2) It determines the therapeutic regimen
(3) It defines the probability of complete remission
(4) It is based in part on retention of villus structures

267. A woman who has trophoblastic disease would be considered a high-risk patient if metastases are present in her

(1) brain
(2) lungs
(3) liver
(4) vagina

268. Indications for instituting single-agent chemotherapy following evacuation of a hydatidiform mole usually include

(1) a rise in HCG titers
(2) a plateau of HCG titers for 3 successive weeks
(3) failure of HCG titers to return to normal 8 weeks after evacuation
(4) appearance of liver or brain metastases

269. Criteria that are especially reliable in determining a patient's response to chemotherapy for gestational trophoblastic disease include

(1) duration of the disease
(2) urine levels of HCG
(3) sites of metastasis
(4) the patient's age

## SUMMARY OF DIRECTIONS

| A | B | C | D | E |
|---|---|---|---|---|
| 1, 2, 3 only | 1, 3 only | 2, 4 only | 4 only | All are correct |

270. Observations on the role of actinomycin D and methotrexate in the management of gestational trophoblastic disease suggest that

(1) resistance to one agent results in cross-resistance to the other
(2) actinomycin D is safer than methotrexate for women whose liver function is impaired
(3) there is no additive effect in combining the two agents
(4) actinomycin D is as effective as methotrexate for primary treatment

271. Choriocarcinoma is characterized by which of the following statements?

(1) It usually metastasizes by hematogenous routes
(2) It is preceded by molar pregnancy in about 85 percent of cases
(3) It can occur several years after a molar pregnancy
(4) It most commonly metastasizes to the liver

272. Which of the following diagnostic procedures can be helpful in establishing the diagnosis of ectopic tubal pregnancy?

(1) Culdoscopy
(2) Laparoscopy
(3) Culdocentesis
(4) Colposcopy

273. True statements about interstitial tubal pregnancy include which of the following?

(1) Its incidence increases in women who have had a salpingectomy
(2) It tends to rupture at an earlier stage than other tubal pregnancies
(3) A significant percentage can be diagnosed before rupture
(4) Rupture causes less blood loss than rupture of pregnancies in the ampullary portion of the tube

**DIRECTIONS**: The group of questions below consists of lettered choices followed by several numbered items. For each numbered item select the **one** lettered choice with which it is **most** closely associated. Each lettered choice may be used once, more than once, or not at all.

**Questions 274-277**

For each clinical history given below, select the diagnosis with which it is most likely to be associated.

(A) Incomplete abortion
(B) Unruptured ectopic pregnancy
(C) Threatened abortion
(D) Persistent corpus luteum cyst
(E) Pelvic inflammatory disease

274. A 22-year-old woman, whose last menstrual period was 5 weeks ago, has had vaginal bleeding for 9 days. She complains of pain in her lower abdomen, especially on the left side. Pelvic examination reveals moderate bleeding from a closed cervical os, a slightly enlarged uterus, and a tenderness in the left adnexa. Pregnancy test is negative

275. A 19-year-old woman, whose last menstrual period was 7 weeks ago, reports that she has had vaginal bleeding for 6 days. In addition, she complains of severe lower abdominal cramps and lightheadedness. Pelvic examination reveals moderate bleeding from a patulous cervix. Pale tissue is noted in the posterior fornix. The uterus is slightly enlarged, and the patient notes mild tenderness in the region of the uterus and adnexa. Pregnancy test is negative

276. A 27-year-old woman, whose last menstrual period was 6 weeks ago, complains of having had vaginal bleeding and right-lower-quadrant pain for the last 2 weeks. Pelvic examination shows slight bleeding from a closed cervix. The uterus seems normal and there is a tender mass, 4 cm square, in the right adnexa. Pregnancy test is negative

277. A 25-year-old woman, whose last menstrual period was 5 weeks ago, says that vaginal spotting with bright red blood and lower abdominal cramps began 5 days ago. Pelvic examination reveals a closed cervix and slight bleeding. The uterus seems normal or slightly enlarged. Pregnancy test is read as doubtful for pregnancy

# Spontaneous Abortion, Ectopic Pregnancies, and Trophoblastic Disease Answers

**253. The answer is D.** *(Reid, p 258.)* A number of investigators have detected a high frequency of chromosomal abnormalities by tissue culture of first trimester abortuses. The frequency of these abnormalities is about 36 percent, of which approximately 45 percent are autosomal trisomies, 25 percent are polyploidies, and 20 percent are 45,XO. The remaining 10 percent include autosomal monosomies, structural abnormalities, and mosaics.

**254. The answer is D.** *(Green, ed 3. pp 290-293.)* The variability in clinical presentation of ectopic tubal pregnancy makes it one of the most difficult diagnostic problems in gynecology. Although tubal disease is an important etiological factor, in most cases the tube is grossly and microscopically normal. Abdominal pain and vaginal bleeding are the most common symptoms. The pain, which is usually colicky and mild at first, later becomes intense and constant. In at least one-quarter of affected women, amenorrhea, which is considered to be characteristic of intrauterine gestation, does not develop. Tubal pregnancies that have "aborted" and become reimplanted are the most common cause of abdominal pregnancies.

**255. The answer is A.** *(Pritchard, ed 16. p 564.)* Injection of a radiopaque substance into the uterine cavity produces a characteristic x-ray picture in a woman who has a hydatidiform mole, which is characterized by the histological transformation of placental villi into vesicles filled with glutinous material as a result of the proliferation of the trophoblast. The etiology of these changes has not been established. The individual hydropic villi are outlined by the dye in the figure accompanying the question, and their grapelike appearance is easily appreciated. As the early clinical course resembles that of a pregnant woman, when symptoms of a mole begin to occur, the woman is often treated for threatened miscarriage until a definitive diagnosis is made (i.e., until the characteristic vesicles are passed). Although no fetal skeleton should be observed in an x-ray of a woman who has a hydatidiform mole unless an intrauterine pregnancy is also present, recent studies have shown that hydatidiform mole has a 46,XX karyotype and have suggested that this chromosomal content is a result of the duplication of the paternal X-carrying haploid without any maternal contribution.

256. **The answer is D.** *(Kistner, ed 3. pp 305-308. Pritchard, ed 16. pp 539-540.)* The clinical history presented in this question is a classic one for a ruptured tubal pregnancy accompanied by a hemoperitoneum. Because pregnancy tests are negative in almost 50 percent of cases, they are of little practical value in an emergency. Dilatation and curettage would not permit rapid enough diagnosis, and the results obtained by this procedure are variable. Posterior colpotomy requires an operating room, surgical anesthesia, and an experienced operator with a scrubbed and gowned associate. Refined optic and electronic systems have improved the accuracy of laparoscopy, but this new equipment is not always available, and the procedure requires an operating room and, usually, surgical anesthesia. Culdocentesis is a rapid, nonsurgical method to confirm the presence of unclotted, intra-abdominal blood from a ruptured tubal pregnancy.

257. **The answer is D.** *(Novak, ed 9. pp 566-570.)* The photomicrograph accompanying the question shows villi within a tubular structure; the villi are easily identified by the presence of cytotrophoblasts. The diagnosis is tubal ectopic pregnancy. Molar pregnancy, incomplete abortion, and missed abortion also can be associated with the presence of villi, but specimens from these disorders would not be obtained at laparotomy.

258. **The answer is E.** *(Mattingly, ed 5. pp 379-380.)* Most authorities believe that the placenta should remain within the abdominal cavity following delivery of an abdominal pregnancy, because removal can lead to blood loss that can be quite difficult to control. If removal of the placenta is desired, it is best to wait until the placental vessels have fibrosed. Some investigators have treated affected women with methotrexate to speed up trophoblastic degeneration. A history of abdominal fetal movements and discomfort suggests abdominal pregnancy, which can be diagnosed by radiography, ultrasonography, failure of oxytocin to induce labor, or other means able to demonstrate the presence of a fetus in the abdomen. Most abdominal pregnancies stem from reimplantation of a ruptured or an aborted early tubal pregnancy.

259. **The answer is E.** *(Mattingly, ed 5. pp 367-370.)* Ectopic pregnancy, which occurs most commonly in the fallopian tubes but also in the ovary, peritoneal cavity, and broad ligament, appears to be more common among black women than white women. The incidence of ectopic pregnancy seems to be increasing (although the mortality rate is decreasing); the incidence is especially high—10 to 20 times that of the general population—in women who have had a previous tubal pregnancy or undergone tubal plastic surgery. Histological evidence of pel-

vic inflammatory disease is found in a significant number of women who have had tubal pregnancies. However, this increase in the incidence of ectopic pregnancy in women who have pelvic inflammatory disease may be due to the antibiotics used to treat the disease, rather than the disease itself.

**260. The answer is D.** *(Novak, ed 9. pp 587-592. Romney, ed 2. pp 1094-1097.)* The history, clinical picture, and tissue sample of the woman described in the question are characteristic of hydatidiform mole. The most common initial symptoms include an enlarged-for-dates uterus and continuous or intermittent bleeding in the first two trimesters. Other symptoms include hypertension, proteinuria, and hyperthyroidism. Hydatidiform mole is ten times as common in the Far East as in North America, and it occurs more frequently in women over 45 years of age. The tissue sample shows a villus with hydropic changes and no vessels. Grossly, these lesions appear as small, clear clusters of grapelike vesicles, the passage of which confirms the diagnosis.

**261. The answer is B.** *(Hilgers, Gynecol Oncol 2:460-475, 1974.)* Ultrasonography is the safest and the most reliable method for early diagnosis of hydatidiform mole. Amniography, although another accurate method, requires percutaneous insertion of a needle into the uterine cavity and injection of a radiopaque contrast dye, which carries a risk of radiation exposure to a normal fetus. An abdominal roentgenogram cannot demonstrate a hydatidiform mole; however, if a fetal skeleton is visualized, it is unlikely that a hydatidiform mole also exists since coexisting molar and fetal pregnancies are rare. Elevated human chorionic gonadotropin (HCG) titers are not diagnostic. Pelvic arteriography would expose an accompanying normal fetus to high doses of radiation.

**262. The answer is A.** *(Hilgers, Gynecol Oncol 2:460-475, 1974.)* The condition of women who have hydatidiform moles but no evidence of metastatic disease should be followed routinely after uterine evacuation by HCG titers. Most authorities agree that prophylactic chemotherapy should not be employed in the routine management of women having hydatidiform moles, because 85 to 90 percent of affected patients will require no further treatment. For a young woman in whom preservation of reproductive function is important, surgery is not routinely indicated.

**263. The answer is E.** *(Rutledge, p 143.)* Adnexal masses are present in approximately one-third of women who have hydatidiform moles. These masses represent theca-lutein cysts that result from human chorionic gonadotropin stimulation. The cysts tend to be bilateral and usually require no therapeutic intervention, unless they undergo torsion, an unusual event.

**264. The answer is A (1, 2, 3).** *(Hilgers, Gynecol Oncol 2:460-475, 1974. Romney, ed 2. pp 1093-1094.)* The term gestational trophoblastic disease refers to a group of neoplasms—that is, hydatidiform mole, choriocarcinoma, and chorioadenoma destruens—that is characterized by the histological degeneration of the gestational trophoblast. Although the pregnancy itself can be affected (e.g., hydatidiform mole), neoplasms of this group also can be diagnosed following normal intrauterine pregnancies, ectopic pregnancies, or abortions. Chorioadenoma destruens is a molar lesion that has invaded the myometrium; choriocarcinoma, which can occur anywhere in the uterus, is composed of malignant trophoblastic cells that metastasize easily. The term gestational trophoblastic disease is preferred because these neoplasms are often managed without a precise histological diagnosis. The presence or absence of metastases is more important in determining prognosis and treatment.

**265. The answer is D (4).** *(Hilgers, Gynecol Oncol 2:460-475, 1974. Romney, ed 2. pp 1093-1094.)* Viable trophoblastic tissue produces HCG; therefore, the presence of elevated HCG titers confirms the amount of functioning trophoblastic tissue and thus the size of the tumor. Monitoring serial HCG titers allows the physician to determine not only the need for chemotherapy but also its effectiveness. Theca-lutein cysts tend to decrease in size following evacuation of a hydatidiform mole despite the persistence of viable trophoblastic cells; and normal cyclic menstruation may reappear in spite of continued disease activity. Chest x-ray changes often persist for several months after HCG titers have returned to normal.

**266. The answer is D (4).** *(Hilgers, Gynecol Oncol 2:460-475, 1974.)* The classification of gestational trophoblastic disease is based both on its histological appearance (including villus-structure retention) as well as on the location of its metastases. This method of classification has not been found to be a reliable indicator of prognosis or management and does not provide a means of estimating the likelihood of complete remission. A better classification distinguishes between metastatic and nonmetastatic gestational trophoblastic diseases as well as between gestational and nongestational trophoblastic diseases, such as primary choriocarcinoma of the ovary.

**267. The answer is B (1, 3).** *(Hilgers, Gynecol Oncol 2:460-475, 1974.)* Women whose trophoblastic disease has metastasized to the brain or liver have poorer prognoses and require more intense treatment than women who have lung or vaginal metastases. The selection of chemotherapeutic regimens is based on this and other prognostic factors; localized radiation therapy frequently is employed to reduce the risk of hemorrhage when brain and liver metastases are present.

**268. The answer is A (1, 2, 3).** *(Hilgers, Gynecol Oncol 2:460-475, 1974. Romney, ed 2. pp 1098-1099.)* Single-agent chemotherapy usually is instituted if levels of HCG have remained elevated 8 weeks after evacuation of a hydatidiform mole. Approximately 50 percent of the patients who have persistently high HCG titers will develop malignant sequelae. If HCG titers rise or reach a plateau for 2 to 3 successive weeks following molar evacuation, single-agent chemotherapy should be instituted, provided that the trophoblastic disease has not metastasized to the liver or brain. The presence of such metastases usually requires initiation of combination chemotherapy.

**269. The answer is A (1, 2, 3).** *(Hilgers, Gynecol Oncol 2:460-475, 1974.)* Women who have had gestational trophoblastic disease for less than 4 months, whose 24-hour urine titers of HCG are less than 100,000 IU, and whose metastases are limited to the vagina or lungs have a 95-percent cure rate and are thus considered low-risk patients. Patients whose disease has lasted for more than 4 months, whose HCG titer is greater than 100,000 IU per 24 hours, and who have liver or brain metastases, on the other hand, are classified as high-risk patients.

**270. The answer is C (2, 4).** *(Hilgers, Gynecol Oncol 2:460-475, 1974.)* The first successful treatment regimen for women who had gestational trophoblastic disease consisted of single-agent methotrexate chemotherapy. Subsequent studies combining methotrexate, actinomycin D, and an alkylating agent were successful in treating methotrexate-resistant trophoblastic disease. Actinomycin D, then studied as a single agent, proved to be as effective as methotrexate; in addition, it was not hampered by cross-resistance in methotrexate-resistant tumors and was safer to use in women who had impaired liver function.

**271. The answer is B (1, 3).** *(Hilgers, Gynecol Oncol 2:460-475, 1974.)* Choriocarcinoma, which is made up of anaplastic and hyperplastic cytotrophoblastic and syncytial constituents, usually metastasizes by hematogenous routes and can produce symptoms caused by metastasis to nonreproductive organs several years following the last known pregnancy. The most common site of distant metastasis is the lung. Approximately 50 percent of choriocarcinomas are preceded by hydatidiform mole; the other 50 percent may have been preceded by abortions, ectopic pregnancies, or even term pregnancies.

**272. The answer is A (1, 2, 3).** *(Wynn, ed 2. p 131.)* Colposcopy is used to examine cervical and vaginal epithelium and would not be helpful in diagnosing a suspected case of ectopic pregnancy. Both culdoscopy and laparoscopy involve the insertion of an endoscope into the peritoneal cavity, the former through the posterior vaginal fornix and the latter through the umbilicus. Either procedure can aid in establishing a diagnosis of ectopic pregnancy. Culdocentesis, the insertion of a needle through the posterior vaginal fornix, can detect a ruptured ectopic pregnancy.

**273. The answer is B (1, 3).** *(Mattingly, ed 5. pp 376-377.)* Rupture of an interstitial tubal pregnancy can cause severe blood loss, because this area is supplied by both uterine and ovarian vessels. Serious shock usually ensues rapidly. Because interstitial tubal pregnancies usually rupture at a later stage than other tubal pregnancies, a significant percentage can be diagnosed before rupture. Women who have had salpingectomies are at increased risk for interstitial pregnancy, and it has been suggested that salpingectomy by too vigorous a cornual wedge resection is the cause.

**274-277. The answers are: 274-B, 275-A, 276-D, 277-C.** *(Kistner, ed 3. pp 305-312. Pritchard ed 16. pp 535-540.)* Vaginal bleeding and lower abdominal pain following a delayed onset of menses can suggest any of the disorders presented. Standard pregnancy tests are rarely positive if onset of menses has been delayed for less than 15 days. Bleeding and cramping accompanied by no other significant symptoms suggest a **threatened abortion**; the presence of tissue and a dilated cervix, on the other hand, points to a diagnosis of **incomplete abortion**. Because symptoms of an **unruptured ectopic pregnancy** and a **persistent corpus luteum cyst** are so similar, the slight enlargement of the uterus that is sometimes associated with the former may be the only way to distinguish the two disorders. Definitive diagnosis of any of these disorders might require laparoscopy. However, with the introduction of the serum pregnancy test which can detect pregnancy as early as 1 week to 10 days after ovulation, virtually all pregnancy episodes (ectopic or otherwise) are detectable. Likewise, culdocentesis is an outpatient procedure that can detect free intra-abdominal blood and can avert a laparoscopy/laparotomy if negative, especially when combined with a negative serum pregnancy test.

# Medical, Surgical, and Obstetrical Complications of Pregnancy

**DIRECTIONS**: Each question below contains five suggested answers. Choose the one best response to each question.

278. A woman who has adult-onset (class B) diabetes requires an elective cesarean section. Her diabetes has been well controlled throughout the pregnancy and she has had normal uterine growth. Her first antepartum visit was at 18 weeks. Weekly oxytocin challenge tests and daily urinary estriol determinations have been within normal limits. It has been decided that the cesarean section should be performed at 38 weeks. Which of the following tests would provide the most useful information on the day prior to the procedure?

(A) Fasting blood glucose
(B) Fetal biparietal diameter
(C) Radiographic study of fetal femoral epiphyses
(D) Lecithin-sphingomyelin ratio
(E) Amniotic fluid alpha-fetoprotein level

279. The initial maternal immunological response to a primary rubella infection is the elaboration of

(A) immunoglobulin M
(B) immunoglobulin G
(C) immunoglobulin A
(D) immunoglobulin D
(E) complement-fixation antibodies

280. Viremia and the presence of rubella virus in the throat of infected individuals bear which of the following relationships to the onset of the rubella rash?

(A) They precede the rash by 5 to 7 days
(B) They precede the rash by 1 to 2 days
(C) They occur coincidentally with the rash
(D) They occur 1 to 2 days after the rash
(E) They bear no consistent relationship to the onset of the rash

281. Although rheumatic heart disease is becoming less common, it still occurs during pregnancy. Deteriorating cardiac status in a pregnant woman is most likely to be associated with

(A) aortic regurgitation
(B) aortic stenosis
(C) mitral regurgitation
(D) mitral stenosis
(E) tricuspid regurgitation

## Questions 282-284

A 24-year-old primigravid woman develops spider angiomata, palmar erythema, and diffuse pruritus at 28 weeks gestation. You obtain a set of liver function tests, which reveal the following serum levels: alkaline phosphatase, 190 IU/L (normal: 21-91 IU/L); glutamic oxaloacetic transaminase, 38 IU/L (normal: 6-18 IU/L); total bilirubin, 1.8 mg/100 ml (normal: 0.3-1.0 mg/100 ml); direct bilirubin, 1.0 mg/100 ml (normal: 0.1-0.3 mg/100 ml).

282. What is the most likely diagnosis of this woman's condition?

(A) Cirrhosis
(B) Infectious hepatitis
(C) Cholestasis
(D) Acute pancreatitis
(E) Cholecystitis

283. The most appropriate treatment would be

(A) observation
(B) bed rest and high-protein diet
(C) oral corticosteroids
(D) low-fat diet
(E) oral cholestyramine

284. After delivery, the physician should advise the woman to

(A) avoid further pregnancies
(B) avoid high-fat foods
(C) avoid oral contraceptives
(D) have a cholecystectomy
(E) none of the above

285. The most common cause of uterine rupture during pregnancy is

(A) previous myomectomy
(B) previous cesarean section
(C) external trauma
(D) transverse lie
(E) oxytocin stimulation of labor

286. In a pregnant woman who has had prolonged, premature rupture of the fetal membranes, the earliest sign of chorioamnionitis would be

(A) maternal fever
(B) maternal leukocytosis
(C) maternal tachycardia
(D) fetal tachycardia
(E) a foul odor to the amniotic fluid

287. Which of the following statements concerning placenta previa is true?

(A) Its incidence decreases with maternal age
(B) Its incidence is unaffected by parity
(C) The initial hemorrhage is painless and rarely fatal
(D) Management no longer includes a "double set-up"
(E) Bleeding is usually painful

288. Which of the following statements describes rupture of a classic cesarean section scar in pregnant women?

(A) It can be prevented by delivery by cesarean section
(B) It is much less likely to occur than rupture of a lower-segment scar
(C) One-third of ruptures occur before the onset of labor
(D) Perinatal mortality rate is 10 percent
(E) Maternal mortality rate is 15 percent

289. All of the following conditions are known to be associated with clinically evident coagulopathies EXCEPT

(A) retained dead fetus
(B) severe pre-eclampsia
(C) sepsis
(D) intra-amniotic prostaglandin $F_{2\alpha}$ abortion
(E) amniotic fluid embolism

290. The most common cause of death in women who have eclampsia is

(A) ruptured liver
(B) acute renal failure
(C) cerebral hemorrhage
(D) pulmonary embolism
(E) septic shock

291. The x-ray shown below reveals which of the following conditions?

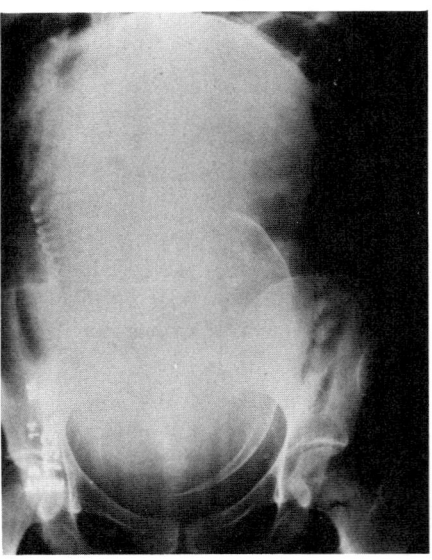

(A) Hydrocephaly
(B) Anencephaly
(C) Fetus papyraceus
(D) Normal breech presentation
(E) Term pregnancy with a dermoid cyst

292. A 32-year-old woman at term develops a clinically obvious coagulopathy following a classic episode of abruptio placentae. Fibrinogen concentrate should NOT be ordered for this woman because

(A) it is commercially unavailable
(B) it carries a risk of hepatitis
(C) it increases the risk of hepatic subcapsular hemorrhage
(D) the patient's primary requirement is platelets
(E) the primary objective should be to stop fibrinolysis

**DIRECTIONS**: Each question below contains four suggested answers of which **one** or **more** is correct. Choose the answer:

| | | | |
|---|---|---|---|
| A | if | 1, 2, and 3 | are correct |
| B | if | 1 and 3 | are correct |
| C | if | 2 and 4 | are correct |
| D | if | 4 | is correct |
| E | if | 1, 2, 3, and 4 | are correct |

293. A 27-year-old woman (gravida 3, para 2) comes to the delivery floor at 37 weeks gestation. She has had no prenatal care. She complains that, on bending down to pick up her 2-year-old child, she experienced sudden, severe back pain. This pain now has persisted for 2 hours. Approximately 30 minutes ago she noted bright red blood coming from her vagina. By the time she arrives at the delivery floor, she is contracting strongly every 3 minutes; the uterus is quite firm even between contractions. By abdominal palpation the fetus is vertex with the head deeply engaged. Fetal heart rate is 130 beats per minute. The fundus is 38 cm above the symphysis. Blood for clotting is drawn, and a clot forms in 4 minutes. Clotting studies are sent to the laboratory. The initial course of action would be to

(1) stabilize maternal circulation
(2) administer oxytocin to stimulate labor
(3) insert an intrauterine catheter for fetal monitoring
(4) administer heparin immediately

294. If polyhydramnios is suspected, which of the following maternal conditions must be ruled out?

(1) Rh isoimmunization
(2) Systemic lupus erythematosus
(3) Diabetes mellitus
(4) Congenital heart disease

295. Premature separation of the placenta occurs more commonly than normal in association with which of the following conditions?

(1) Previous abruptio placentae
(2) Chronic hypertension
(3) Pregnancy-induced hypertension
(4) Delivery of twins

296. Common findings in the incompetent cervix syndrome include

(1) painless dilatation of the cervix
(2) a history of cervical trauma
(3) spontaneous rupture of the membranes at midpregnancy
(4) recurrent miscarriage at 14 to 16 weeks gestation

297. Birth of twins is associated with an increased incidence of

(1) prolapsed cord
(2) pre-eclampsia
(3) velamentous cord insertion
(4) hydramnios

## SUMMARY OF DIRECTIONS

| A | B | C | D | E |
|---|---|---|---|---|
| 1, 2, 3 only | 1, 3 only | 2, 4 only | 4 only | All are correct |

298. True statements about pregnancy-induced hypertension include which of the following?

(1) The incidence varies widely around the world
(2) Women who have had hypertension of pregnancy once have a 10-percent chance of developing it in a later pregnancy
(3) Elevations in systolic or diastolic blood pressures may be diagnostically significant even at blood pressure values less than 140/90 mm Hg
(4) Young primiparous women have the lowest incidence

299. Pregnancy-induced hypertension is associated with which of the following lesions?

(1) Periportal hemorrhages
(2) Ischemic lesions
(3) Large subcapsular hematomas
(4) Primary fibrin deposits in hepatic arterioles

300. In infected women, cytomegalovirus can be recovered from

(1) saliva
(2) urine
(3) cervical secretions
(4) liver biopsy specimens

301. Nausea and vomiting are common in pregnancy. Hyperemesis gravidarum, however, is a much more serious and potentially fatal problem. Findings that shoud alert the physician to the diagnosis of hyperemesis gravidarum **early** in its course include

(1) electrocardiographic evidence of hypokalemia
(2) weight loss
(3) jaundice
(4) ketonuria

302. Erythroblastosis fetalis can be caused by maternal incompatibility with which of the following fetal erythrocyte antigens?

(1) Kell
(2) Kidd
(3) Duffy
(4) Lewis

303. True statements about appendicitis during pregnancy include which of the following?

(1) Premature labor occurs commonly
(2) Mortality rate is much higher in pregnant than nonpregnant women
(3) Symptoms may be mistaken for those classically associated with pregnancy itself
(4) It is frequently mistaken for pyelitis of the right kidney

304. A 29-year-old Rh-negative woman (gravida 5, para 4) is 18 weeks pregnant. Her last child had erythroblastosis fetalis and required four exchange transfusions at birth. The father of her current pregnancy is not the father of her other children. Although he is Rh positive, he is a heterozygote. True statements regarding this case include which of the following?

(1) The infant has a 75-percent chance of being born with erythroblastosis fetalis
(2) The woman should be followed with serum titers, and amniocentesis should be performed when the titers are two dilutions greater than baseline values
(3) If fetal hydrops is demonstrated ultrasonographically or amniographically, intrauterine transfusions should be performed prior to 20 weeks gestation
(4) O-negative blood that has been crossmatched against the mother's serum should be used for an intrauterine transfusion, if a transfusion is indicated

305. Ovarian neoplasms of pregnant women can be characterized by which of the following statements?

(1) They are usually malignant
(2) They are most often confined to one ovary
(3) They may spread transplacentally to the fetus
(4) They can be mistaken for a cystic corpus luteum

306. Pregnant women who have diabetes mellitus are affected more often than nondiabetic women by which of the following conditions?

(1) Pre-eclampsia and eclampsia
(2) Infection
(3) Postpartum hemorrhage after vaginal delivery
(4) Hydramnios

307. True statements about hypoparathyroidism in pregnancy include which of the following?

(1) Its etiology is most commonly iatrogenic
(2) It is best treated with oral calcium and vitamin D
(3) It is a contraindication to breast-feeding
(4) It is associated with a marked increase in spontaneous abortions

308. Maternal hyperparathyroidism can be characterized by which of the following statements?

(1) Diagnosis is made more often after pregnancy than during pregnancy
(2) Neonatal tetany may result
(3) Incidence of pathological fractures is increased
(4) Fertility, labor, and delivery are adversely affected

| SUMMARY OF DIRECTIONS | | | | |
|---|---|---|---|---|
| A | B | C | D | E |
| 1, 2, 3 only | 1, 3 only | 2, 4 only | 4 only | All are correct |

309. True statements about hyperthyroidism in pregnancy include which of the following?

(1) Affected women may be treated with thiourea compounds
(2) It is harder to control in pregnant than in nonpregnant women
(3) It may cause neonatal thyrotoxicosis
(4) It is an indication for interrupting a pregnancy

310. Hypothyroidism can be characterized by which of the following statements?

(1) It is uncommon during pregnancy
(2) It is associated with an increased abortion rate
(3) It is associated with an increased stillbirth rate
(4) It is generally improved by pregnancy

311. Women who have systemic lupus erythematosus should be counseled that

(1) pregnancy is contraindicated, because it will exacerbate the disease
(2) if pregnant, they should have a therapeutic abortion to prevent a progression of their symptoms
(3) their disease is likely to inhibit their fertility
(4) their disease is likely to flare up after delivery

312. Systemic lupus erythematosus is associated with which of the following?

(1) High abortion rate
(2) High stillbirth rate
(3) High prematurity rate
(4) Higher-than-normal female-to-male ratio among liveborn siblings

313. Pregnancy has which of the following effects on a diabetic woman?

(1) Tendency toward ketoacidosis during early pregnancy
(2) Tendency toward hyperglycemia during early pregnancy
(3) Increase in insulin requirement during early pregnancy
(4) Increase in insulin requirement during late pregnancy

314. Pregnancy should be strongly discouraged in women who have

(1) atrial septal defect
(2) ventricular septal defect
(3) patent ductus arteriosus
(4) Eisenmenger's syndrome

## Questions 315-318

For each description that follows, select the microorganism with which it is most likely to be associated.

(A) Rubella virus
(B) Cytomegalovirus
(C) Group A β-hemolytic streptococci
(D) Group B β-hemolytic streptococci
(E) *Toxoplasma gondii*

315. This organism may cause epidemics of puerperal sepsis

316. A pregnant woman may become infected with this organism by contact with infected cat feces

317. An effective vaccine exists for the prevention of adult infection with this organism

318. This organism is an important cause of neonatal sepsis and meningitis

## Questions 319-321

For each clinical situation that follows, select the most likely placental disorder.

(A) Placenta accreta
(B) Placenta circumvallata
(C) Placenta membranacea
(D) Placenta succenturiata
(E) Vasa praevia

319. A 24-year-old woman, gravida 2, para 1, goes into premature labor at 33 weeks gestation after an apparently normal antepartum course

320. An apparently normal pregnancy culminates in the spontaneous delivery of an infant who weighs 3.2 kg (7 lb) with Apgars 9/9. The placenta delivers spontaneously followed by an unusual amount of uterine bleeding

321. After the low forceps delivery of an infant who weighs 1.8 kg (4 lb) to a 27-year-old woman, gravida 4, para 3 (whose second baby was born by cesarean section due to fetal distress but whose third baby delivered vaginally), the placenta does not deliver spontaneously. After 20 minutes the obstetrician attempts a manual removal but is unable to identify a plane of cleavage

## Questions 322-326

For each description that follows, select the disorder with which it is most likely to be associated.

(A) Placental polyps
(B) Placenta previa
(C) Abruptio placentae
(D) Ectopic pregnancy
(E) Spontaneous abortion

322. Associated with the Arias-Stella phenomenon

323. Premature placental separation

324. Associated with maternal hypertension

325. May be due to defective vascularization of the decidua caused by inflammation or atrophy

326. Usually accompanied by thickened placental villi, hemorrhage into the decidua basalis, and evidence of necrosis in tissues near the bleeding

## Questions 327-329

For each patient described, choose the diagnostic category (according to the Priscilla White classification) that is most appropriate.

(A) Normal
(B) Class A diabetic
(C) Class B diabetic
(D) Class C diabetic
(E) Class D diabetic

327. The patient is a 17-year-old primigravid woman who was diagnosed as being diabetic at age 9 and is currently taking 30 units of Lente insulin every morning. She is 18 weeks pregnant

328. The patient is a 26-year-old woman, gravida 3, para 2. Her first baby weighed 3.9 kg (8.6 lb) and her second baby weighed 4.1 kg (9 lb). A glucose tolerance test is done at 28 weeks gestation after 2 days of carbohydrate loading; the test dose is 100 g of oral glucose. Blood sugars (mg/100 ml) are measured as follows: fasting, 88; 1-hour, 179; 2-hour, 144; 3-hour, 123

329. The patient is a 22-year-old primigravid woman who has a strong family history of diabetes. About 6 months before becoming pregnant, she had a glucose tolerance test. Although test results were abnormal, she was told that the results indicated chemical diabetes only and that no treatment was necessary. She has never been in ketoacidosis and has no symptoms now. An oral glucose tolerance test given at 28 weeks gestation (same method as described in question 328) reveals the following levels (mg/100 ml): fasting value, 92; 1-hour, 170; 2-hour, 148; 3-hour, 127

# Medical, Surgical, and Obstetrical Complications of Pregnancy

# Answers

**278. The answer is D.** *(Villee, p 193.)* The major problem associated with elective cesarean sections is the development of the respiratory distress syndrome in a premature infant. Pulmonic maturation may be delayed in infants of mothers who have chemical or adult-onset diabetes. Although femoral epiphyseal studies and measurement of the biparietal diameter might confirm the dates, only the lecithin-sphingomyelin ratio can give some assurance of pulmonic maturity. The maternal fasting blood sugar level, though it may reflect the development of neonatal hypoglycemia, is not as crucial in the clinical situation of this question as the lecithin-sphingomyelin ratio.

**279. The answer is A.** *(Burrow, p 421.)* The first response to a primary infection of rubella and other viruses is the elaboration of immunoglobulin M (IgM). Although IgM, once produced, is present for at least several weeks, rising levels of immunoglobulin G (IgG) account for the fact that IgG eventually comprises nearly all antibody detected in the serum. Complement-fixation antibodies usually appear 7 to 10 days after appearance of the rubella rash.

**280. The answer is A.** *(Burrow, p 417.)* Both viremia and the excretion of virus from the throats of individuals infected with rubella occur 5 to 7 days before the appearance of the characteristic maculopapular rash. The importance of this relationship is that by the time a pregnant woman first notes the appearance of a rash on one of her children, she already has been exposed to the disease and may, in fact, be infected. If one member of a family develops rubella, all other members who are susceptible to the disease usually become infected.

**281. The answer is D.** *(Burrow, pp 110-115.)* Nearly all of the circulatory changes that normally accompany pregnancy are harmful to a woman who has mitral stenosis. Left atrial pressure rises because of increased cardiac output and shortened diastolic filling time; as a result, pulmonary flow is accentuated. Atrial fibrillation may occur suddenly during pregnancy, and pulmonary edema may supervene. Cardioversion may be necessary to reverse atrial fibrillation. Mitral regurgitation is unlikely to be worsened by pregnancy, although prophylaxis for subacute bacterial endocarditis would be indicated for affected women. Aortic stenosis is unusual as a pure lesion; associated problems, if they are going to develop at all, are most likely to develop in the immediate postpartum period, when rapid volume shifts can occur. Aortic regurgitation also is rare as a pure lesion and again is most likely to cause problems just after delivery.

**282-284. The answers are: 282-C, 283-E, 284-C.** *(Pritchard, ed 16. pp 757-759.)* The most likely diagnosis for the woman described in the question is cholestatic jaundice of pregnancy (cholestasis). Spider angiomata and palmar erythema are normal occurrences in pregnant women and do not imply hepatic disease. Generalized pruritus in pregnancy, however, may be caused by cholestasis. In this disorder, bilirubin may or may not be elevated; and elevation, if present, is usually mild. Although serum alkaline phosphatase levels may double during normal pregnancy, they are usually even higher in cholestasis of pregnancy. If placental (heat-stable) alkaline phosphatase can be distinguished from the hepatic isozyme, then hepatic alkaline phosphatase will show an increase in patients with cholestasis. Levels of serum glutamic-oxaloacetic transaminase may be mildly elevated.

The appropriate treatment for this condition, if the itching is intractable, is oral cholestyramine, an exchange resin that ties up bile salts in the gastrointestinal tract and presumably reduces their levels in the periphery. Although its safety in pregnancy is not unequivocally established, oral cholestyramine is commonly used for this condition when treatment is necessary.

Cholestasis tends to recur in subsequent pregnancies and to accompany use of oral contraceptives. If the patient is willing to go through another pregnancy with the symptoms described, it is not contraindicated; however, oral contraceptives are probably a poor choice for family planning in these patients. In the case described, there is no reason to suspect pancreatitis; cirrhosis is not exacerbated by pregnancy; the enzyme values do not support hepatitis; and the patient does not show symptoms of cholecystitis.

**285. The answer is B.** *(Pritchard, ed 16. pp 861-863.)* More than any other factor, delivery by cesarean section in an earlier pregnancy predisposes a woman to uterine rupture in subsequent pregnancies. Oxytocin stimulation of labor also is associated with rupture of the uterus and, in fact, may be the second most common cause. Other factors associated less frequently with uterine rupture include previous myomectomy, external trauma (such as an accident or bullet wound), breech delivery, and congenital or acquired defects of the uterus.

**286. The answer is D.** *(Monif, p 297.)* Fetal tachycardia in a woman who has had prolonged, premature rupture of fetal membranes strongly suggests chorioamnionitis—a bacterial infection of the fetal membranes that is confirmed by stain and culture of amniotic fluid. Maternal fever and leukocytosis are later signs of infection. The presence of fetal tachycardia should be interpreted with caution, however, because it also can arise as a result of an arrhythmia or exposure to drugs, such as atropine.

**287. The answer is C.** *(Pritchard, ed 16. pp 513-514.)* The initial hemorrhage in placenta previa is usually painless and rarely fatal. If a fetus is premature and if hemorrhaging is not severe, vaginal examination of a woman suspected of having placenta previa frequently can be delayed until 37 weeks of gestation; this delay in the potentially hazardous examination reduces the risk of prematurity, which often is associated with placenta previa. Vaginal examination, when needed to determine whether a low-lying placenta is covering the internal os of the cervix, should be performed in an operating room fully prepared for an emergency cesarean section (i.e., a "double set-up"). Increasing maternal age and multiparity are associated with a higher incidence of placenta previa.

**288. The answer is C.** *(Pritchard, ed 16. p 863.)* Rupture of a classic cesarean section scar is several times more likely than rupture of a scar of the lower uterine segment. Because one-third of ruptures of a classic scar occur before the onset of labor (sometimes as much as several weeks before term), cesarean section delivery cannot prevent such ruptures. Rupture of a classic scar is associated with a perinatal mortality rate of approximately 50 percent; the maternal mortality rate, however, is usually no higher than 5 percent.

**289. The answer is D.** *(Ratnoff, p 175.)* Retention of a dead fetus can be associated with the slow release of thromboplastic material into the peripheral circulation. Amniotic fluid embolism, on the other hand, causes a dramatic and rapid intravascular coagulopathy. Disseminated intravascular coagulation caused by sepsis probably results from the exposure of subendothelial collagen to circulating blood. Severe pre-eclampsia can be associated with markedly depressed platelet counts as well as diffuse fibrin deposition in multiple small vessels. Although saline abortions have been implicated in causing disseminated intravascular coagulation, prostaglandin $F_{2\alpha}$ abortions thus far have not.

**290. The answer is C.** *(Burrow, pp 68-69. Romney, ed 2. p 688.)* Pre-eclampsia, a disease of pregnancy, is characterized by hypertension, edema, and proteinuria after the 20th week of gestation. If not properly treated, pre-eclampsia may progress to eclampsia with accompanying convulsions and coma. Cerebral hemorrhage is the most common cause of death in women who have eclampsia. Sixty percent of women who die 2 days or less after the onset of convulsions are found subsequently to have cerebral hemorrhages. Evidence suggests that the pathophysiology of the lesions involves cerebral vasoconstriction. The maternal mortality rate from eclampsia is 3 to 5 percent; the fetal mortality rate is 17 to 20 percent.

**291. The answer is A.** *(Pritchard, ed 16. pp 824-826.)* The three criteria for an x-ray diagnosis of hydrocephaly in utero are a small face in relation to a large head, a hydrocephalic head that is usually globular instead of ovoid, and an often scarcely visible or very thin shadow of a hydrocephalic cranium. In the x-ray accompanying the question, the tremendous disproportion between head and body leaves little doubt as to the diagnosis of hydrocephaly.

**292. The answer is B.** *(Beck, ed 2. pp 326-327, 562-565. Ratnoff, p 175.)* Fibrinogen concentrate is obtained from pooled plasma. Compared to a unit of whole blood, it is approximately 30 times more likely to cause hepatitis. Fibrinogen delivered in whole blood, cryoprecipitate, or fresh frozen plasma carries much less risk of hepatitis. Women who have disseminated intravascular coagulation following a placental abruption are more in need of fibrinogen than platelets. Primary fibrinolysis is almost never a contributing factor to the coagulopathies of these women.

**293. The answer is B (1, 3).** *(Pritchard, ed 16. pp 495-508. Romney, ed 2. pp 675-676.)* The patient described in the question presents with a classic history for abruption—that is, the sudden onset of abdominal pain accompanied by bleeding. Physical examination reveals a firm, tender uterus with frequent contractions, which confirms the diagnosis. The fact that a clot forms within 4 minutes suggests that coagulopathy is not present. Because abruption is often accompanied by hemorrhaging, it is important that appropriate fluids (i.e., lactated Ringer's solution and whole blood) be administered immediately to stabilize the mother's circulation. Cesarean section may be necessary in the case of a severe abruption, but only when fetal distress is evident or delivery is unlikely to be accomplished vaginally. Internal monitoring equipment should provide an early warning that the fetus is compromised. The internal uterine catheter provides pressure recordings, which are important if oxytocin stimulation is necessary. Generally, however, patients with abruptio placentae are contracting vigorously and do not need oxytocin.

**294. The answer is B (1, 3).** *(Pritchard, ed 16. pp 578-579.)* Polyhydramnios is defined as the presence of more than 2000 ml of amniotic fluid. This volume of amniotic fluid results in a tense uterus with a size greater than expected with a left mentoposterior position (LMP) and a fetus that is difficult to outline on palpation. Twin pregnancies (especially monozygotic twins), maternal diabetes mellitus, Rh isoimmunization or any other cause of erythroblastosis fetalis, and congenital anomalies of the fetus, especially gastrointestinal and central nervous system anomalies, are all associated with an increased incidence of polyhydramnios. There is no increased association with maternal systemic lupus erythematosus (SLE) or maternal heart disease.

**295. The answer is E (all).** *(Pritchard, ed 16. pp 495-508.)* Premature separation of the placenta (abruptio placentae) occurs in approximately 1 percent of all deliveries. Previous abruptio placentae, chronic hypertension, and pregnancy-induced hypertension all predispose to premature separation of the placenta. The placenta also is more likely than normal to separate between the birth of a first and second twin. Clinically, the severity of abruption ranges from a minimal amount of vaginal bleeding and rapid labor to massive hemorrhage, shock, consumptive coagulopathy, and fetal death. Clinical signs of abruption include an irritable, tender uterus, an enlarging uterus, hypertonic labor, and abdominal pain. Vaginal bleeding may or may not be present; in fact, some of the most severe abruptions with coagulopathies occur with "concealed hemorrhage," in which the retroplacental clot is contained within the uterus and has no egress to the vagina.

**296. The answer is A (1, 2, 3).** *(Pritchard, ed 16. pp 598-601.)* When an incompetent cervix is suspected, weekly cervical examinations beginning at 16 to 18 weeks gestation can reveal evidence of cervical dilatation or effacement in time to perform corrective surgery. The most commonly used techniques are the Shirodkar cervical suture (cerclage), in which the purse-string suture is buried under the vaginal mucosa and the bladder pushed back for higher placement of the stitch, and the McDonald cervical suture, a simple purse-string suture most widely used when the cervix is well effaced. Once the diagnosis has been made, a cerclage procedure may be performed prophylactically in subsequent pregnancies, prior to any change in the cervix. This is best done at 14 to 16 weeks, well past the time when spontaneous abortion is common. Because it is not until 16 to 18 weeks that the fetus begins to occupy the lower uterine segment, it would be unlikely that incompetent cervix would be the cause of recurrent pregnancy loss at 14 to 16 weeks.

**297. The answer is E (all).** *(Benirschke, NY State J Med 61:4499, 1961. Robertson, Obstet Gynecol 23:330, 1964.)* In one series of 450 twins, the incidence of cord prolapse was 3 percent for the first twin and 5 percent for the second; the overall hospital incidence was 1 percent during the same period of time. In the same series the incidence of pre-eclampsia in mothers of twins was reported to be 32 percent. Twins also have a greatly increased incidence of velamentous cord insertion and therefore are at risk for rupturing a vasa praevia. Hydramnios has been reported to occur in 12.5 percent of twins.

**298. The answer is B (1, 3).** *(Burrow, pp 75-76.)* Worldwide, the incidence of pregnancy-induced hypertension varies from a low of 2 percent in the Far East to almost 30 percent in Puerto Rico. Peak incidences occur in two groups: young primiparous women and multiparous women who are older than 35 years of age. Moreover, women who have had hypertension of pregnancy in the past have a 33-percent chance of developing the disease again in later pregnancies. Because of the difficulty in defining normal blood pressures for pregnant women, elevations in the systolic component of 20 mm Hg or more or the diastolic component of 10 mm Hg or more during pregnancy are defined as abnormal, notwithstanding the absolute blood pressure values. The terminology regarding hypertension in pregnancy is still in flux. The most inclusive term is hypertensive states of pregnancy. This is recommended by the American College of Obstetrics and Gynecology Committee on Terminology for general use. If the hypertension was not present preconception, then pregnancy-induced hypertension is also acceptable, but the term toxemia has fallen into disfavor.

**299. The answer is A (1, 2, 3).** *(Burrow, p 68. Romney, pp 687-688.)* Pregnancy-induced hypertension is associated with two types of hepatic lesions: periportal hemorrhages, which eventually are supplanted by fibrin deposits, and ischemic lesions, which can vary greatly in size and severity. It has been hypothesized that it is the spasm of hepatic arterioles, and not the primary deposition of fibrin, that is responsible for the hemorrhagic lesions.

**300. The answer is E (all).** *(Burrow, p 426.)* Cytomegalovirus can be recovered from the urine, saliva, cervical secretions of infected women, and specimens from a liver biopsy. Urine is the best source for recovering cytomegalovirus, which may be present in concentrations as high as 1 million virus particles per milliliter. Cultures of the virus, which is slow-growing, may not be positive until a month or more has passed.

**301. The answer is C (2, 4).** *(Burrow, pp 285-292.)* Hyperemesis gravidarum is intractable vomiting of pregnancy and is associated with disturbed nutrition. Early signs of the disorder include weight loss, up to 5 percent of body weight, and acetonuria. Because vomiting causes potassium loss, electrocardiographic evidence of potassium depletion, such as inverted T waves and prolonged Q-T and P-R intervals, is usually a later finding. Jaundice also is a later finding and is probably due to fatty infiltration of the liver; occasionally acute hepatic necrosis occurs. Hypokalemic nephropathy with isosthenuria may occur late. Hypoproteinemia also may result, caused by poor diet as well as by albuminuria. Patients who have hyperemesis gravidarum are best treated (if the disease is early in its course) with parenteral fluids and electrolytes, sedation, rest, vitamins, and antiemetics if necessary. In some cases, isolation of the patient is necessary. Very slow reinstitution of oral feeding is permitted after dehydration and electrolyte disturbances are corrected. Therapeutic abortion may be necessary in rare instances; usually, however, the disease improves spontaneously as pregnancy progresses.

**302. The answer is A (1, 2, 3).** *(Pritchard, ed 16. pp 972-973.)* Erythroblastosis fetalis, also known as isoimmune hemolytic disease of the newborn, results from the transplacental passage of maternal blood-group antibodies and subsequent destructive reaction with fetal erythrocyte antigens. It is theoretically possible for any blood-group antigen with the exceptions of Lewis and I antigens to cause erythroblastosis fetalis. Lewis and I antigens are not present on fetal red blood cells; furthermore, the antibodies to these two antigens are immunoglobulin M, which does not cross the placenta.

**303. The answer is E (all).** *(Mattingly, ed 5. pp 409-413.)* Pregnancy and appendicitis share many of the same signs and symptoms, including nausea, vomiting, abdominal discomfort, constipation, and leukocytosis. Because urinary tract symptoms are associated commonly with appendicitis of pregnant women, the disease also can be mistaken for pyelitis. Maternal mortality rates and fetal prematurity are increased in women who are pregnant and have appendicitis.

**304. The answer is D (4).** *(Queenan, ed 2. pp 12-14, 27-44, 149-267.)* An Rh-negative woman married to a heterozygous Rh-positive man has a 50-percent chance of having an Rh-positive baby. Spectrophotometric analyses of the woman's amniotic fluid should be performed to detect bilirubin pigment; they should begin at 22 to 23 weeks gestation and be repeated every 2 weeks until delivery. (Serum titers are very inaccurate in women who were sensitized in previous pregnancies.) If the level of bilirubin pigment suggests imminent fetal demise, intrauterine transfusion of the pulmonically immature fetus is indicated. Transfusion before 23 to 24 weeks gestation should not be attempted because of technical difficulties and the extremely poor chance of success at so early a stage. When intrauterine transfusions are performed, O-negative blood that is crossmatched against the mother's serum should be used.

**305. The answer is C (2, 4).** *(DiSaia, pp 188-189.)* Ovarian neoplasms associated with pregnancy are usually benign; only 3 to 6 percent are found to be malignant. The neoplasms are most often unilateral when malignant. It has been estimated that 10 percent of ovarian masses discovered during pregnancy represent an enlarged, cystic corpus luteum. Transplacental spread of ovarian carcinoma to the fetus has not been documented.

**306. The answer is E (all).** *(Pritchard, ed 16. p 743.)* Maternal diabetes mellitus can affect a pregnant woman and her fetus in many ways. The development of pre-eclampsia or eclampsia is about four times as likely as among nondiabetic women. Infection also is more likely not only to occur but also to be severe. The incidences of fetal macrosomia or death and of dystocia are increased; and hydramnios is common. The likelihood of postpartum hemorrhage after vaginal delivery and the frequency of cesarean section both are increased in diabetic women.

**307. The answer is A (1, 2, 3).** *(Burrow, pp 268-271.)* Hypoparathyroidism is most commonly iatrogenic, occurring when the parathyroid glands have been inadvertently removed at the time of thyroidectomy. The disease is characterized by low levels of serum calcium and high levels of serum phosphate. The usual treatment is oral calcium and vitamin D. Hypoparathyroid mothers should not breast-feed their children, because the calcium drain of breast-feeding may worsen their hypocalcemia. The outcome of pregnancy in the hypoparathyroid patient who is under treatment should be excellent. If tetany occurs during pregnancy, hypoparathyroidism should be suspected, especially if the patient has had previous thyroid surgery; the most common cause of tetany during pregnancy, however, is alkalosis.

**308. The answer is A (1, 2, 3).** *(Burrow, pp 265-268.)* Hyperparathyroidism, which often is caused by a parathyroid adenoma, is characterized by elevated levels of serum calcium and symptoms associated with hypercalcemia. These symptoms include weakness, nausea, polyuria, and polydipsia; renal stones and pathological fractures also can occur. Because the milder of these symptoms may be seen in normal pregnancies, the presence of hyperparathyroidism may be missed during pregnancy. More than half of the infants born to hyperparathyroid mothers have neonatal tetany—the first clue, in many instances, to the fact that the mother has the disease. The tetany is due to hypocalcemia in the newborn and occurs usually at 5 to 14 days of age. Hyperparathyroid patients do not have increased infertility problems. Labor and delivery are usually normal; however, the incidence of small-for-dates infants is increased.

**309. The answer is B (1, 3).** *(Burrow, pp 226-236.)* Hyperthyroidism in pregnancy may cause neonatal thyrotoxicosis. The mechanism is not the transmission of triiodothyronine or thyroxine to the baby, but rather the crossing of long-acting thyroid stimulator (LATS) to the baby with subsequent hyperfunction of the fetal thyroid gland. Not all hyperthyroid women have LATS; and it is only those who do who are at risk for neonatal thyrotoxicosis. The usual treatment for hyperthyroidism in pregnancy is administration of thiourea compounds, although in some centers surgery is popular. Hyperthyroidism often becomes less severe during pregnancy, especially during the last trimester, at which time requirements for thiourea drugs often decrease. Because hyperthyroidism is a treatable disorder, it is not an indication for terminating a pregnancy.

**310. The answer is A (1, 2, 3).** *(Burrow, pp 213-216.)* It is not known why hypothyroidism is uncommon during pregnancy; however, the most widely supported explanation is that many hypothyroid patients are anovulatory and thus do not easily become pregnant. However, if a hypothyroid patient does become pregnant, her disease, if untreated, could lead to abortion and stillbirth. For this reason, most perinatologists prefer to treat hypothyroidism vigorously during pregnancy. For example, if a woman who has been placed on low-dose thyroid replacement for poorly documented hypothyroidism becomes pregnant, administration of thyroid hormone probably should be increased to full replacement dose for the remainder of the pregnancy; after delivery, hormone therapy should be discontinued in order to re-evaluate thyroid function.

**311. The answer is D (4).** *(Burrow, pp 786-794. Pritchard, ed 16. pp 768-769.)* Studies of the effect of pregnancy on the course of systemic lupus erythematosus (SLE) have been inconsistent in their findings. Some studies suggest a worsening of the disease, while others show remission or no effect at all. If a woman who is informed that her lupus might get worse during pregnancy still wants to have a child, she may be supported in her plans. Women should be advised to await a clinical remission of the disease before attempting pregnancy, since the course of SLE is more favorable when pregnancy occurs during such a remission. In most cases therapeutic abortion is not indicated, because the postpartum flare-up, especially in renal disease, may occur whether the pregnancy has been terminated by abortion or delivery. For some very sick patients, however, abortion may be lifesaving. Only in cases involving severe renal disease does lupus seem to decrease the fertility rate.

**312. The answer is E (all).** *(Burrow, p 790.)* The incidence of spontaneous abortion is about 40 percent after the clinical onset of systemic lupus erythematosus. If renal disease is present, the abortion rate is higher still. Prematurity has been found to be present in as many as one-third of deliveries, and stillbirths occur with increased frequency. The sex ratio also is changed in the offspring of women who have lupus erythematosus, with a decrease in the ratio of liveborn males to total liveborn siblings. The preponderance of females with lupus may, in fact, be due to the high mortality rate among male siblings antenatally.

**313. The answer is D (4).** *(Burrow, pp 179-180.)* Although during early pregnancy the diabetogenic effects of placental hormones are not marked, there is still a net transfer of glucose from mother to fetus. For this reason, there is a tendency toward maternal hypoglycemia rather than hyperglycemia; ketoacidosis is rare and insulin reactions are common. In fact, one of the first symptoms of pregnancy in a diabetic woman may be hypoglycemia and decreasing insulin need. Later on in pregnancy, however, insulin requirements increase markedly and are about two-thirds higher than before pregnancy. Hypoglycemia now becomes less of a problem than ketoacidosis.

**314. The answer is D (4).** *(Burrow, pp 120-127.)* Eisenmenger's syndrome consists of severe pulmonary hypertension combined with a bidirectional or reversed shunt through a patent ductus arteriosus or an atrial or ventricular septal defect. The death rate during pregnancy for women who have this syndrome is higher than in any other form of congenital heart disease. Death usually occurs at or just after delivery and is probably associated with a sudden drop in peripheral vascular resistance. Atrial and ventricular septal defects, in the absence of pulmonary hypertension and right-to-left shunting, rarely cause problems during pregnancy. Unless shunting is minimal, a patent ductus arteriosus is usually detected by the time a woman becomes pregnant. Again, only reversal of the shunt should pose any problems.

**315-318. The answers are: 315-C, 316-E, 317-A, 318-D.** *(Monif, pp 73, 197-198, 306, 455.)* Group A β-hemolytic streptococci can cause puerperal or postoperative pelvic infection. Outbreaks of puerperal fever are still reported on obstetrical services, though not at anywhere near the frequency of 50 years ago. When the disease does occur, a point source among the hospital personnel should be suspected.

Group B β-hemolytic streptococci, which also can cause puerperal fever, have recently been recognized as a major cause of severe neonatal infection. The organism can be isolated from the cervices of about 5 percent of all pregnant women; infection of the infant, which can result in sepsis, occurs as the infant passes through the vagina.

*Toxoplasma gondii*, a protozoan parasite, is transmitted by flies from cat feces to human food. Thus, humans can become infected by consuming infected meat that is inadequately cooked or by coming in direct contact with feces of an infected cat. Acute toxoplasmosis in a pregnant woman may cause a fulminant fetal infection; infected neonates may be born with microcephaly, intracranial calcification, or other symptoms.

An effective attenuated-virus vaccine is available for immunization against rubella. However, its use is contraindicated for pregnant women and commonly is associated with development of arthralgia in adults.

**319-321. The answers are: 319-B, 320-D, 321-A.** *(Pritchard, ed 16. pp 134, 551, 553, 574, 575, 884-888.)* A circumvallate placenta contains a grayish-white ring located a variable distance from the edge of the placenta. The membranes (amnion and chorion) are folded over at this ring and are not in contact with the substance of the placenta peripheral to the ring. The fetal vessels do not go beyond the ring. Placenta circumvallata is associated with an increased rate of prematurity; why the rate is increased is unknown.

A succenturiate placenta is characterized by an accessory lobe apart from the main body of the placenta. Fetal vessels usually course through the membranes between the main and accessory lobes and can be identified on inspection of the membranes. If the fetal vessels on their way between the lobes should pass over the cervix, vasa praevia occurs. This condition is potentially dangerous, because the membranes may rupture, in turn rupturing a fetal vessel and causing fetal hemorrhage. If a succenturiate lobe is left within the uterus after the main body of the placenta has been delivered, postpartum hemorrhage can result; therefore, the presence of an accessory lobe should be checked for by intrauterine exploration.

Placenta accreta is a condition in which the usual plane of cleavage (Nitabuch's layer) between the placenta and decidua is absent and the villi attach to the myometrium. It is more common in women who have uterine scars, such as in the patient described in the question, and who had undergone previous cesarean section. Complications of placenta accreta are in part iatrogenic. An overly vigorous attempt at manual removal may cause uterine inversion or perforation and severe bleeding. A hysterectomy may be necessary, although leaving the placenta in place and treating the patient with methotrexate may suffice. Severe complications are most common with the more severe forms of placenta accreta. These forms are known as placenta increta, if the villi grow into the muscle of the uterus, and placenta percreta, if the placenta grows through the myometrium.

**322-326. The answers are: 322-D, 323-C, 324-C, 325-B, 326-E.** *(Pritchard, ed 16. pp 495-498, 508-510, 529-530, 588-594.)* Placenta previa is characterized by defective vascularization of the decidua, secondary to either inflammatory or atrophic changes; in this uncommon condition, the placenta is implanted over or near the internal os. Abruptio placentae (placental abruption), which is associated very closely with maternal hypertension, is the premature separation of the placenta from the uterus. The Arias-Stella phenomenon, which refers to certain changes of the glands and epithelium of the endometrium, frequently is associated with ectopic pregnancy; however, this phenomenon also can occur whenever a conceptus is blighted and may be seen in intrauterine as well as extrauterine pregnancies. Spontaneous abortions histologically are accompanied by distended placental villi, hemorrhage into the decidua basalis, and evidence of necrotic changes in the region surrounding the hemorrhage.

**327-329. The answers are: 327-E, 328-A, 329-B.** *(Burrow, pp 177-179.)* The Priscilla White classification is the most widely used descriptive categorization of diabetes in pregnant women. To a certain extent, as the classes progress alphabetically, the fetal prognosis becomes increasingly poor. A class A diabetic patient is one who either is diagnosed during pregnancy and needs no insulin or, if diagnosed before pregnancy, was asymptomatic and needed no treatment. A class B diabetic patient is overtly diabetic and was diagnosed after the age of 20; in addition, the duration of the disease is less than 10 years. A class C diabetic woman was diagnosed either between the ages of 10 and 20 years or from 10 to 20 years ago. Diagnosis of a class D diabetic woman was made either before the age of 10 or more than 20 years ago.

The normal values for a glucose tolerance test during pregnancy differ from those of nonpregnant women. With 2 days of carbohydrate loading and a 100 g oral glucose tolerance test, a patient, to be considered diabetic, must exceed two of the following four blood-sugar values (mg/100 ml): fasting, 90; 1-hour, 165; 2-hour, 145; 3-hour, 125. If serum or plasma levels are measured, the standards are 14 percent higher.

# Diagnosis and Management of Disorders of Labor, Delivery, and Puerperium

**DIRECTIONS**: Each question below contains five suggested answers. Choose the **one best** response to each question.

330. The graph below depicts a labor curve for a woman, gravida 2, para 1, with intact membranes. This labor curve is compatible with which of the following conditions?

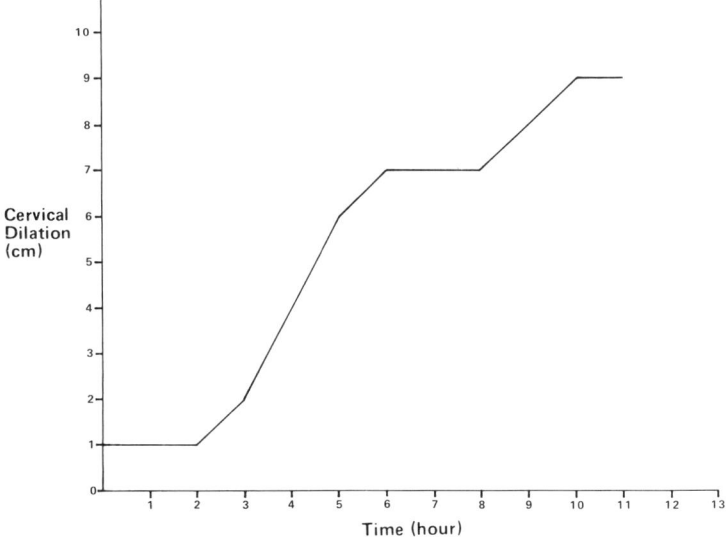

(A) Normal labor
(B) Protracted latent phase
(C) Protracted active phase
(D) Primary dysfunction
(E) Hypertonic dysfunction

331. The fetal monitoring strip shown below demonstrates which of the following?

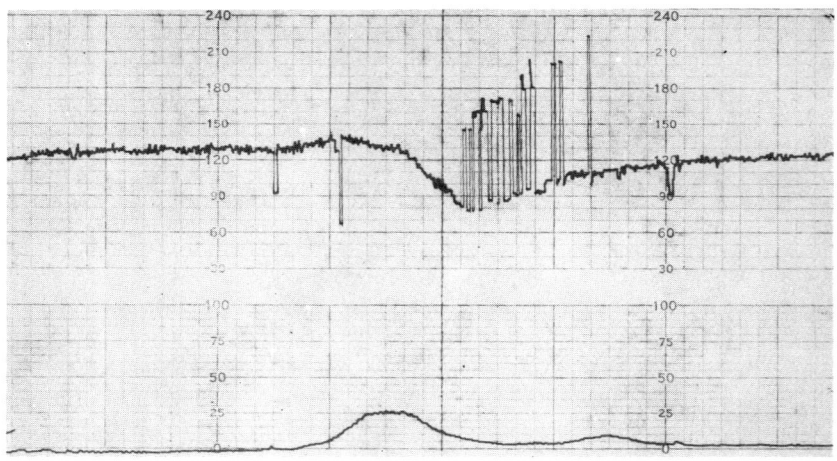

(A) A uteroplacental insufficiency pattern
(B) A cord pattern
(C) Head compression
(D) Uneventful labor
(E) Fetal death

332. Beta sympathomimetic drugs, which can inhibit uterine activity, include all of the following EXCEPT

(A) salbutamol
(B) ritodrine
(C) propranolol
(D) terbutaline
(E) fenoterol

333. Late deceleration patterns (type II dips) on a fetal monitoring strip represent

(A) cord compression
(B) pulmonary immaturity
(C) fetal hypoxia secondary to decreased perfusion of the intervillous spaces
(D) congenital cardiac conduction defects
(E) entry of the fetal head into the pelvic brim

## Questions 334-335

A 24-year-old primigravid woman, who is intent on breast-feeding, decides upon a home delivery. Immediately after the birth of a 4.1-kg (9-lb) infant, the patient bleeds massively due to extensive vaginal and cervical lacerations. She is brought in shock to the nearest hospital. Nine units of blood are transfused over 2 hours, and the blood pressure returns to a reasonable level. A hemoglobin value the next day is 7.5 g/100 ml, and 3 units of packed red blood cells are given.

334. The most likely late sequela to consider in this woman would be

(A) hemochromatosis
(B) Stein-Leventhal syndrome
(C) Sheehan's syndrome
(D) Simmonds' syndrome
(E) Cushing's syndrome

335. Development of this sequela could be evident as early as

(A) 6 hours postpartum
(B) 1 week postpartum
(C) 1 month postpartum
(D) 6 months postpartum
(E) 1 year postpartum

## Questions 336-337

A woman develops endometritis after a cesarean section has been performed. She is treated with penicillin and gentamicin but fails to respond.

336. Which of the following bacteria is resistant to these antibiotics and is likely to be responsible for this woman's infection?

(A) *Proteus mirabilis*
(B) *Bacteroides fragilis*
(C) *Escherichia coli*
(D) Alpha streptococci
(E) Anaerobic streptococci

337. The treatment of choice for this woman's condition would be

(A) polymyxin
(B) ampicillin
(C) cephalothin
(D) vancomycin
(E) clindamycin

## Obstetrics and Gynecology

**DIRECTIONS:** Each question below contains four suggested answers of which **one** or **more** is correct. Choose the answer:

| | | | |
|---|---|---|---|
| A | if | 1, 2, and 3 | are correct |
| B | if | 1 and 3 | are correct |
| C | if | 2 and 4 | are correct |
| D | if | 4 | is correct |
| E | if | 1, 2, 3, and 4 | are correct |

338. Agents that are currently approved in the United States by the Food and Drug Administration specifically for inhibition of premature labor include

(1) ethanol
(2) isoxsuprine
(3) terbutaline
(4) ritodrine

339. Fetal presenting positions that are usually undeliverable vaginally include

(1) brow
(2) mentum anterior
(3) mentum posterior
(4) left sacrum posterior

340. Precipitate labor, which most often occurs in multiparous women, is associated with a greater-than-normal incidence of which of the following?

(1) Amniotic fluid embolism
(2) Fetal hypoxia
(3) Fetal cerebral trauma
(4) Cervical laceration

341. Hypertonic dysfunctional labor generally can be expected to

(1) cause little pain
(2) occur in the active phase of labor
(3) react favorably to oxytocin stimulation
(4) respond to sedation

342. A genital tract infection after delivery (puerperal infection) is characterized by which of the following statements?

(1) A temperature of $38°C$ ($100.4°F$) or higher on any 2 of the first 10 postpartum days (excluding the first day) is considered the standard definition of puerperal morbidity
(2) Iatrogenic causes are significant sources of infection
(3) The most common pathogens involved are those that normally inhabit the bowel and lower genital tract
(4) Anaerobic infections are common and frequently are caused by *Bacteroides, Peptostreptococcus,* or *Clostridium*

343. Following a vaginal delivery, a woman develops a fever, lower abdominal pain, and uterine tenderness. She is alert, and her blood pressure and urine output are good. Large gram-positive rods suggestive of *Clostridia* are seen in a smear of the cervix. Management should include

(1) close observation for renal failure or hemolysis
(2) immediate radiographic examination for gas in the uterus
(3) high-dose antibiotic therapy
(4) hysterectomy

344. A 25-year-old woman has recently delivered a 4-kg (8½-lb) boy and is now experiencing heavy vaginal bleeding. The obstetrician should rule out which of the following causes of postpartum hemorrhage?

(1) Uterine atony
(2) Vaginal/cervical lacerations
(3) Retained placental fragments
(4) Blood dyscrasias

345. Chorioamnionitis develops in a woman whose membranes have ruptured at 35 weeks gestation; the fetus is alive. Management should include

(1) systemic antibiotics
(2) high-dose corticosteroids
(3) delivery by either a brief induction or cesarean section
(4) heparinization

346. Barton forceps can be described by which of the following statements?

(1) It is useful when the fetal head is in a transverse position in a platypelloid pelvis
(2) It is useful when traction and rotation are to be performed simultaneously
(3) Application of the blades can be adjusted by a sliding lock
(4) The posterior blade is hinged

347. Predisposing factors to face presentation include

(1) contracted pelvis
(2) pendulous abdomen
(3) anencephalic fetus
(4) large fetus

**DIRECTIONS:** The groups of questions below consist of lettered choices followed by several numbered items. For each numbered item select the **one** lettered choice with which it is **most** closely associated. Each lettered choice may be used once, more than once, or not at all.

## Questions 348-350

For each of the following clinical descriptions, select the procedure that would be most appropriate.

(A) External version
(B) Internal version
(C) Midforceps rotation
(D) Low transverse cesarean section
(E) Classic cesarean section

348. A 24-year-old primigravid woman, at term, has been in labor for 16 hours and has been 9 cm dilated for 3 hours. The fetal vertex is in the right occiput posterior position, at +1 station, and molded. There have been mild late decelerations for the last 30 minutes. Twenty minutes ago, the fetal scalp pH was 7.27; it is now 7.20

349. A 24-year-old woman (gravida 3, para 2) is at 40 weeks gestation. The fetus is in the transverse lie presentation

350. You have just delivered an infant weighing 2.5 kg (5.5 lb) at 39 weeks gestation. Because the uterus still feels large, you do a vaginal examination. A second set of membranes is bulging through a fully dilated cervix, and you feel a small part presenting in the sac. A fetal heart is auscultated at 60 beats per minute

## Questions 351-354

For each clinical situation described below, choose the appropriate type of obstetrical forceps.

(A) Simpson forceps
(B) Kielland forceps
(C) Barton forceps
(D) Chamberlen forceps
(E) Piper forceps

351. A breech delivery with an aftercoming head

352. The occiput transverse position in a flat pelvis

353. Fetal rotation

354. An elective low forceps delivery

# Diagnosis and Management of Disorders of Labor, Delivery, and Puerperium

# Answers

**330. The answer is C.** *(Pritchard, ed 16. pp 385-387, 787-789.)* The labor described by the curve is characteristic of a protracted active phase. That the woman has entered the active phase is evident by the rate of dilatation (from 2 cm to 7 cm) over the space of 3 hours. The normal active phase progresses at a rate of at least 1.5 cm/hr in a multiparous woman and 1.2 cm/hr in a nulliparous woman. After 7 cm dilatation is reached in this patient, however, progress slows down to 2 cm over the next 4 hours, or 0.5 cm/hr, and the active phase is said to be protracted. Another name for this condition is secondary arrest of labor. (Primary arrest of labor is arrest of progress before the active phase has begun.) If this woman's contractions are adequate by intrauterine monitoring and further progress does not occur, most obstetricians would perform a cesarean section. If hypotonic dysfunction were causing the protracted labor, some obstetricians would stimulate contractions with intravenous oxytocin.

**331. The answer is A.** *(McCrann, Clin Perinatol 1:242, 1974.)* The fetal monitoring strip that accompanies the question illustrates a uteroplacental insufficiency pattern. In this pattern, deceleration of the heart rate begins after the onset of the contraction, and the lowest rate occurs after the contraction has peaked. In addition there is a very slow return to the baseline. This is an ominous pattern and implies significant fetal hypoxia. Scalp pH sampling is warranted in this situation; and if acidosis is present and the pattern persists with subsequent contractions, rapid delivery should be performed. Diabetes mellitus and hypertensive states of pregnancy are diseases that typically compromise the functional capacity of the placenta.

**332. The answer is C.** *(Ingemarsson, Am J Obstet Gynecol 125:520, 1976.)* Beta-stimulating drugs have been used succesfully to inhibit uterine activity. Drugs of this type, such as fenoterol, ritodrine, salbutamol, and terbutaline, stimulate $\beta_2$ receptors of the uterus; cardiac $\beta_1$ receptors are also stimulated but only to a minor degree. Propranolol is a beta-blocking agent.

**333. The answer is C.** *(Hon, p 102.)* Late deceleration patterns on a fetal monitoring strip result from fetal hypoxia caused by decreased perfusion, during contractions, of the intervillous spaces. A healthy fetus can tolerate the transient hypoxia resulting from contractions without exhibiting heart rate changes. Thus, late deceleration patterns are ominous, because they indicate that a fetus has very little reserve. Permanent damage of the central nervous system can result if the hypoxia is allowed to persist.

**334-335. The answers are: 334-C, 335-B.** *(Pritchard, ed 16. pp 879-880.)* A disadvantage of home delivery is the lack of facilities to control postpartum hemorrhage. The woman described in the question delivered a large baby, suffered multiple soft-tissue injuries, and went into shock, needing 9 units of blood by the time she reached the hospital. Sheehan's syndrome seems a likely possibility in this woman. This syndrome of anterior pituitary necrosis related to obstetrical hemorrhage can be diagnosed by 1 week postpartum, as lactation fails to commence normally. Although many modern women choose hormonal therapy to prevent lactation, the woman described in the question was intent on breast-feeding and so would not have received suppressant. She therefore could have been expected to begin lactation at the usual time. Other symptoms of Sheehan's syndrome include amenorrhea, atrophy of the breasts, and loss of thyroid and adrenal function.

The other presented choices for late sequelae are rather far-fetched. Hemochromatosis would not be expected to occur in this healthy young woman, especially since she did not receive prolonged transfusions. Cushing's, Simmonds', and Stein-Leventhal syndromes are not known to be related to postpartum hemorrhage.

It is important to note that home delivery is **not** a predisposing factor to postpartum hemorrhage.

**336. The answer is B.** *(Monif, pp 8, 439-441.)* Infections caused by *Bacteroides fragilis*, a gram-negative anaerobic bacillus, are a significant obstetrical problem. Not only is the organism resistant to many commonly used antibiotics (including penicillin and gentamicin), but it is difficult to isolate, culture, and identify as well. The high incidence of gynecological and obstetrical *B. fragilis* infections may be due to the pathogen's predominance among the anaerobic bacteria of the lower bowel. Although the other organisms listed in the question also can cause postpartum infection, they are sensitive to antibiotic therapy with penicillin and gentamicin.

**337. The answer is E.** *(Monif, pp 8, 441-442.)* Clindamycin is the most effective antibiotic for treating women who have bacteroidosis. Chloramphenicol and tetracycline are alternative choices for antibiotic therapy in nonpregnant women; however, tetracycline-resistant strains of *Bacteroides fragilis* may be emerging. Lincomycin and erythromycin also can be effective in the management of affected women.

**338. The answer is D (4).** *(Barden, Obstet Gynecol 56:1-6, 1980.)* Although all the drugs listed in the question have been shown to successfully inhibit uterine activity, only ritodrine has been approved by the Food and Drug Administration for use in the treatment of preterm labor. This approval came in 1980 after worldwide experience with the drug had proven very favorable; in fact, ritodrine is expected to become the treatment of choice for premature labor in the next decade. Studies with ritodrine have shown it to be at least as useful as terbutaline or isoxsuprine with a minimum incidence of maternal hypotension noted. However, when using ritodrine, particularly if corticosteroids are administered concomitantly to accelerate fetal pulmonary maturity, care must be taken not to overload the patient with fluids and to be vigilant for early signs of pulmonary edema. This complication has been reported within the range of intake volumes that the healthy pregnant female could otherwise handle without difficulty. At present, the pathophysiology of this condition remains ill-defined.

**339. The answer is B (1, 3).** *(Pritchard, ed 16. pp 812-813.)* In brow presentation, the fetal head is midway between flexion and extension. Except with an extremely small baby, engagement cannot occur unless flexion to vertex or extension to face presentation supervenes. In face presentation, delivery is by flexion rather than extension as in vertex presentations. Only the mentum anterior is capable of flexing under the pubic symphysis. The mentum posterior position does not allow flexion, because the neck is too short to go around the sacrum. The left sacrum posterior position is a variation of breech presentation. Although many present-day obstetricians would rarely deliver a breech vaginally, the breech presentation is by no means undeliverable.

**340. The answer is E (all).** *(Pritchard, ed 16. pp 793-795.)* Precipitate labor is labor that either is extremely rapid or is not perceived by the patient or obstetrician. For example, some women who have had presacral neurectomy do not have painful contractions and thus may be unaware they are in labor. Rapid precipitate labor, which is more common, may be due to extremely strong or prolonged contractions. Because these contractions interfere with the proper oxygenation of fetal blood, fetal hypoxia can result. Extremely strong or long contractions coupled with an unyielding cervix or vagina may predispose to amniotic fluid embolism or tears of the cervix or vagina. Sudden delivery with rapid compression and decompression of the fetal head may cause cerebral trauma.

**341. The answer is D (4).** *(Pritchard, ed 16. p 792.)* Hypertonic uterine dysfunction is characterized by a lack of coordination of uterine contractions, possibly caused by disorganization of the contraction gradient, which normally is greatest at the fundus and least at the cervix. This type of dysfunction usually appears during the latent phase of labor and is responsive to sedation, not oxytocin stimulation. The disorder is accompanied by a great deal of discomfort with little cervical dilatation (the familiar and painful false labor). After being sedated for a few hours, affected women usually awaken in active labor.

**342. The answer is E (all).** *(Pritchard, ed 16. pp 893-904.)* The agents most responsible for puerperal infections are those normally found in the lower genital tract or in the bowel. These agents may be anaerobic bacteria (most commonly *Bacteroides, Peptostreptococcus,* and *Clostridium*) or aerobic bacteria (such as *Escherichia coli, Klebsiella, Pseudomonas,* and *Enterobacter*); infections caused by a combination of two or more pathogens occur frequently. Most puerperal infections are wound infections; trauma before or during delivery and iatrogenic bacterial contamination are significant etiological factors. Puerperal morbidity is defined as a temperature of 38°C (100.4°F) or higher occurring on any 2 of the first 10 postpartum days, excluding the first.

**343. The answer is A (1, 2, 3).** *(Monif, pp 435-438.)* *Clostridia* can be seen in 5 to 10 percent of pelvic cultures. When the organism is found, appropriate antibiotic therapy (e.g., with penicillin) and close observation for gas gangrene, hemolysis, and renal failure are in order. Presumed identification on the basis of Gram stain alone or the presence of a mild infection without signs of sepsis or extrauterine involvement is not reason enough to proceed to hysterectomy.

**344. The answer is E (all).** *(Pritchard, ed 16. pp 878-879.)* Undoubtedly the most common cause of postpartum hemorrhage in the early puerperium is uterine atony, but vaginal lacerations and retained placental fragments must also be considered. Once these three major causes of hemorrhage have been ruled out, disorders of the coagulation system, either congenital (e.g., von Willebrand's disease) or acquired (e.g., disseminated intravascular coagulation), should be considered. The initial assessment of the woman described in the question should include a determination of previous bleeding problems, time since delivery,

Disorders of Labor, Delivery, and Puerperium 155

special problems encountered during delivery (e.g., manual removal of the placenta or vaginal laceration), quantity of blood loss, vital signs (including positional effect on blood pressure), and uterine consistency. Further diagnostic or therapeutic steps would depend upon this initial assessment of causative factors.

**345. The answer is B (1, 3).** *(Monif, pp 297-299.)* The main mode of treatment for women who have chorioamnionitis is delivery. If the cervix is effaced and dilated, a brief induction could be undertaken; if the cervix is unripe, then abdominal delivery would be in order. Administration of potent antibiotics is important to prevent the development of sepsis in the mother. Although corticosteroids are not indicated in the treatment of women who have uncomplicated chorioamnionitis, such therapy might be valuable if septic shock develops. The use of steroids to accelerate pulmonary maturity would be inappropriate. Heparinization is not indicated in uncomplicated chorioamnionitis. Coagulation disorders, which may be a complication of severe infection, should not be treated unless there is uncontrollable bleeding.

**346. The answer is B (1, 3).** *(Pritchard, ed 16. p 1053.)* A special feature of Barton forceps is the hinged anterior blade. This type of forceps is useful when the fetal head is in a transverse position in a platypelloid pelvis; it should not be used, however, to perform simultaneous traction and rotation. Application of the forceps is by moving the hinged blade about the occiput or face; adjustment is made by a sliding lock.

**347. The answer is E (all).** *(Pritchard, ed 16. pp 809-811.)* Face presentations occur in approximately 0.2 percent of deliveries. A large or anencephalic fetus, contracted pelvis, and pendulous abdomen all make extension of the head more likely. In addition, tumors of the anterior neck or multiple coils of umbilical cord around the neck may predispose to face presentation. Cesarean section commonly is necessary with face presentations; it may be avoided in many cases, however, if the decision is put off until the second stage of labor, when flexion or rotation to the mentum anterior position may occur.

**348-350. The answers are: 348-D, 349-A, 350-B.** *(Pritchard, ed 16. pp 645, 813-817, 1045-1046, 1081-1082, 1093-1095. Romney, ed 2. p 669.)* A woman who has been 9 cm dilated for 3 hours is experiencing a secondary arrest in labor. Deteriorating fetal condition (as evidenced, for example, by late decelerations and falling scalp pH) dictates immediate delivery. A forceps rotation would be inappropriate, because the cervix is not fully dilated. Cesarean section would be the safest and most expeditious method. Classic cesarean section is rarely used now because of greater blood loss and a higher incidence in subsequent pregnancies of rupture of the scar prior to labor. The best procedure would be a low transverse cesarean section.

A transverse lie is undeliverable vaginally. One treatment option is to do nothing and hope that the lie will be longitudinal by the time labor commences. The only other appropriate maneuver would be to perform an external cephalic version. This maneuver should be done in the hospital, with monitoring of the fetal heart. If the version is successful and the cervix is ripe, it might be best to take advantage of the favorable vertex position by rupturing the membranes at that point and inducing labor.

According to some studies, 25 percent of twins are diagnosed at the time of delivery. Although, sonography or radiography can diagnose multiple gestation early in pregnancy, these methods are not used routinely in all medical centers. The second twin is probably the only remaining situation where internal version is permissible. Although some obstetricians might perform a cesarean section for a second twin presenting as a footling or shoulder, fetal bradycardia dictates that immediate delivery be done; and internal podalic version is the quickest procedure.

**351-354. The answers are: 351-E, 352-C, 353-B, 354-A.** *(Pritchard, ed 16. pp 1041-1063, 1070-1075.)* Piper forceps were designed specifically for the delivery of the after-coming head in a vaginal breech delivery. They should never be applied until the head has fully entered the maternal pelvis and is engaged.

Barton forceps are designed for a transverse arrest in a platypelloid (flat) pelvis. The pelvic curve of the forceps is in an appropriate position vis-à-vis the maternal pelvis when the forceps are applied to the occiput transverse. Descent is then accomplished in this position, and rotation to the occiput anterior does not occur until the pelvic floor is reached. Rotation in the midplane thus is unnecessary; indeed, such rotation would be difficult in a flat pelvis.

Kielland forceps are designed specifically for rotation. They have very little pelvic curve and thus are unlikely to cause maternal soft-tissue injury during rotation. They can be used for occiput posterior or transverse positions, in which rotation is planned before traction is applied.

Simpson forceps are the prototype forceps for the molded head. They are useful for low forceps deliveries, and some obstetricians use Simpson or similar forceps for various rotation maneuvers.

Chamberlen forceps, the first true obstetrical forceps, were in use in the late sixteenth century.

# CLINICAL GYNECOLOGY

# Menstrual and Endocrine Disorders

DIRECTIONS: Each question below contains five suggested answers. Choose the one best response to each question.

355. For postmenopausal women in whom cystic glandular hyperplasia of the endometrium has been diagnosed by fractional dilatation and curettage, the usual management is

(A) hysterectomy
(B) hysterectomy preceded by radiation
(C) hysterectomy followed by radiation
(D) hysterectomy and bilateral salpingo-oophorectomy
(E) observation

356. The Sertoli-cell-only syndrome is characterized by which of the following levels of follicle-stimulating hormone (FSH), luteinizing hormone (LH), or both?

(A) Increased FSH levels
(B) Decreased FSH levels
(C) Increased LH levels
(D) Decreased LH levels
(E) Normal FSH and LH levels

357. A 19-year-old man is seen because of late onset of puberty. The laboratory reports the man has azoospermia; and physical and historical findings indicate that he also has a poorly developed sense of smell. The most likely diagnosis is

(A) panhypopituitarism
(B) Reifenstein's syndrome
(C) Klinefelter's syndrome
(D) Kallman's syndrome
(E) Turner's syndrome

358. Amenorrhea can be associated with all of the following conditions EXCEPT

(A) hematometra
(B) uterus didelphys
(C) testicular feminization
(D) Turner's syndrome
(E) Sheehan's syndrome

359. A 35-year-old woman presents with hypotension, cold intolerance, amenorrhea, waxy skin with multiple fine wrinkles, loss of axillary and pubic hair, and loss of skin pigmentation. Her urine sodium levels are normal. The most likely diagnosis is

(A) hypothyroidism
(B) Addison's disease
(C) panhypopituitarism
(D) malignant melanoma
(E) diabetes insipidus

360. In pituitary failure, the usual order of appearance of clinical deficiencies of the tropic hormones is

(A) somatotropin, thyrotropin, corticotropin, prolactin, gonadotropin
(B) thyrotropin, corticotropin, prolactin, gonadotropin, somatotropin
(C) corticotropin, prolactin, gonadotropin, somatotropin, thyrotropin
(D) prolactin, gonadotropin, somatotropin, thyrotropin, corticotropin
(E) gonadotropin, somatotropin, thyrotropin, corticotropin, prolactin

361. A 22-year-old woman (gravida 0) has oligomenorrhea, hirsutism, and fertility problems. Neither muscle mass nor clitoral size is increased. Androgen-production rates are elevated, and ovarian biopsy shows stromal hyperplasia and follicular cells at all stages of development. The most likely diagnosis is

(A) Turner's syndrome
(B) Stein-Leventhal syndrome
(C) Kallman's syndrome
(D) Reifenstein's syndrome
(E) adrenogenital syndrome

362. All of the following statements concerning the postpill amenorrhea syndrome are true EXCEPT that

(A) spontaneous resolution of the amenorrhea frequently occurs
(B) it occurs in approximately 1 percent of women who have taken oral contraceptives
(C) it is usually associated with a normal menstrual history prior to use of oral contraceptives
(D) the treatment of choice is clomiphene
(E) it is associated with normal thyroid function

**DIRECTIONS:** Each question below contains four suggested answers of which **one** or **more** is correct. Choose the answer:

| A | if | 1, 2, and 3 | are correct |
|---|---|---|---|
| B | if | 1 and 3 | are correct |
| C | if | 2 and 4 | are correct |
| D | if | 4 | is correct |
| E | if | 1, 2, 3, and 4 | are correct |

363. Recurring catamenial pneumothorax—a rare disorder of young women—can be described by which of the following statements?

(1) It usually is due to pleural endometriosis
(2) It can be inhibited by ovulation suppression
(3) It occurs with equal frequency on both sides of the chest
(4) It rarely is associated with underlying pulmonary pathology

364. Development of endometrial hyperplasia has been associated with

(1) perimenopausal anovulation
(2) prolonged postpartum anovulation
(3) granulosa-theca-cell tumors
(4) Stein-Leventhal syndrome

365. Asherman's syndrome is characterized by which of the following?

(1) Biphasic basal body temperatures
(2) Diagnosis by endometrial biopsy
(3) Amenorrhea
(4) Remission after removal of an intrauterine device

366. Endometrial dysfunctional bleeding includes which of the following types?

(1) Estrogen breakthrough bleeding
(2) Estrogen withdrawal bleeding
(3) Progesterone breakthrough bleeding
(4) Progesterone withdrawal bleeding

367. Signs or symptoms commonly associated with anorexia nervosa but NOT with hypopituitarism include

(1) marked wasting
(2) loss of axillary and pubic hair
(3) elevated levels of human growth hormone
(4) decreased thyroid activity

368. Mammary-gland development is a common feature of patients who have

(1) testicular feminization
(2) Reifenstein's syndrome
(3) Klinefelter's syndrome
(4) Turner's syndrome

369. The causes of panhypopituitarism include

(1) postpartum hemorrhage
(2) Hand-Schüller-Christian disease
(3) temporal arteritis
(4) empty-sella syndrome

Menstrual and Endocrine Disorders 161

370. An 18-year-old woman has primary amenorrhea. Her growth and development have been normal. Workup of this woman should include

(1) serum FSH and LH levels
(2) karyotype
(3) serum prolactin levels
(4) an endometrial biopsy

371. A 19-year-old woman consults you because of amenorrhea and galactorrhea of 1 year's duration. Her periods previously had been regular. She has had no other symptoms except for a mild headache. Diagnoses compatible with the findings on the CAT scan shown below include

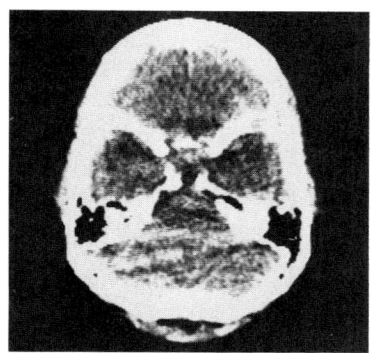

(1) empty-sella syndrome
(2) amenorrhea of a nonpituitary etiology
(3) microadenoma of the pituitary gland
(4) suprasellar lesion of a pituitary adenoma

372. True statements concerning anorexia nervosa include which of the following?

(1) It is seen predominantly in females, rarely in males
(2) Most affected patients have an obsessive-compulsive personality
(3) Mean 24-hour concentration of cortisol is twice normal
(4) Thyroid hormones are in the normal range

373. True statements regarding the empty-sella syndrome include which of the following?

(1) Headache is a common complaint
(2) Most affected patients have visual field defects
(3) It is most commonly seen in middle-aged, obese women
(4) X-ray of the sella turcica often reveals asymmetrical enlargement

374. Primary dysmenorrhea can be characterized by which of the following statements?

(1) Onset is usually with or shortly after menarche
(2) Pelvic examination is usually normal
(3) Irritability and depression are frequent emotional symptoms
(4) Symptoms are related to the release of prostaglandins in the menstrual fluid

## Obstetrics and Gynecology

**DIRECTIONS:** The groups of questions below consist of lettered choices followed by several numbered items. For each numbered item select the **one** lettered choice with which it is most closely associated. Each lettered choice may be used once, more than once, or not at all.

### Questions 375-378

For each case history that follows, select the type of menstrual bleeding with which it most likely is associated.

(A) Progesterone breakthrough bleeding
(B) Progesterone withdrawal bleeding
(C) Estrogen breakthrough bleeding
(D) Estrogen withdrawal bleeding
(E) None of the above

375. A 24-year-old nulligravid woman is being evaluated for infertility. Her cycles are irregular, lasting from 30 to 90 days. Menstrual flow is usually heavy. She also has increasing hirsutism and obesity

376. A 55-year-old woman, 3 years postmenopause, is bothered by hot flashes. Her doctor orders conjugated estrogens (Premarin), 1.25 mg daily for 21 to 28 days. On the fourth month of Premarin therapy, the woman has heavy menstrual flow from the 25th to the 28th day

377. An 18-year-old woman complains of severe dysmenorrhea. She has regular periods every 28 days, with light flow on the first day, heavy flow on the second and third days, and light spotting on the fourth day

378. A 33-year-old woman is placed on one of the low-dose birth-control pills. Two weeks later, having taken nine of the birth-control pills, she calls your office because she has begun to have menstrual flow

### Questions 379-383

For each description that follows, select the type of sexual precocity with which it is most likely to be associated.

(A) True sexual precocity
(B) Incomplete sexual precocity
(C) Isosexual precocious pseudopuberty
(D) Heterosexual precocious pseudopuberty
(E) Precocity due to gonadotropin-producing tumors

379. Defined by the presence of virilizing signs in girls

380. Characterized by the presence of premature adrenarche, pubarche, or thelarche

381. Can arise from cranial tumors or hypothyroidism

382. Stems from premature activation of the hypothalamus-pituitary system

383. Frequently caused by ovarian tumors

# Menstrual and Endocrine Disorders Answers

**355. The answer is E.** *(Rutledge, pp 112-113.)* Cystic glandular hyperplasia progresses to endometrial carcinoma in only 1 to 2 percent of cases. Although some physicians consider it a precursor to adenocarcinoma, cystic hyperplasia is usually thought to antecede adenomatous hyperplasia, which then progresses to endometrial carcinoma in 5 to 15 percent of cases. For most patients, observation is the appropriate mode of management.

**356. The answer is A.** *(Williams, ed 5. pp 328-329.)* The Sertoli-cell-only syndrome is characterized by an increase in follicle-stimulating hormone (FSH) levels; luteinizing hormone (LH) levels remain normal. There are two major theories to explain how the testis controls FSH production. One is the "inhibin" theory, in which the germinal epithelium is thought to produce a water-soluble, nonsteroid substance that regulates FSH secretion. The other theory states that Sertoli cells secrete a steroid, possibly $\Delta^5$-pregnenolone, that controls FSH production. In a testis containing only Sertoli cells, there would be no regulation on, hence no negative feedback of, FSH; therefore, FSH levels would be elevated.

**357. The answer is D.** *(Speroff, ed 2. pp 118, 242.)* The man described in the question has Kallman's syndrome, which is a combination of hypogonadotropic eunuchoidism and hyposmia (an abnormally decreased sense of smell). Whether these two symptoms share a common etiology is not known. Panhypopituitarism and Reifenstein's and Klinefelter's syndromes all can lead to hypogonadism, but none are associated with abnormalities in the sense of smell. Turner's syndrome is gonadal dysgenesis in an individual who has a 45,XO karyotype.

**358. The answer is B.** *(Speroff, ed 2. pp 107-115.)* Didelphia (double uterus) develops due to failure of müllerian structures to fuse in the midline. The endometrium is normal, and menstruation usually occurs from both uteri and both cervices. Hematometra—the accumulation of blood in the uterus—results from cervical stenosis; no blood flows out of the cervix, although the endometrium has normal shedding. Individuals who have testicular feminization have no uterus, thus making menstruation impossible. Women who have Turner's syndrome have nonfunctional ovaries; their amenorrhea is of the hypergonadotropic, hypoestrogenic variety. Certain forms of Turner's syndrome mosaicisms, however, are associated with normal menstruation. Amenorrhea in Sheehan's syndrome is caused by the absence of FSH and LH production by the pituitary gland. Hence, the ovaries are not stimulated to produce estrogen and, as a result, normal menstruation does not occur.

**359. The answer is C.** *(Williams, ed 5. pp 55-59.)* The most likely diagnosis of the woman described in the question is panhypopituitarism. The associated hypotension results from a decrease in cortisone production, which is caused by a lack of corticotropin. Because the adrenal glands still maintain the ability to produce aldosterone, sodium levels are usually unchanged. Cold intolerance, amenorrhea, and changes in skin appearance and pigmentation are frequent signs of hypopituitarism. A patient who has hypothyroidism generally would present with different symptoms from those described, although cold intolerance may be encountered. A patient with Addison's disease would not be able to maintain body sodium. Malignant melanoma causes none of the presenting features described; and although diabetes insipidus may be a symptom of hypopituitarism, it does not cause the described symptomatology.

**360. The answer is E.** *(Williams, ed 5. p 56.)* In pituitary failure, the tropic hormones usually disappear in the following order: gonadotropin, somatotropin, thyrotropin, corticotropin, and prolactin. When all the tropic hormones are gone, the diagnosis of pituitary failure is easy; however, in the evaluation of possible incipient pituitary failure, the sequential disappearance of these hormones can be an important diagnostic clue. Thus, a woman who develops amenorrhea followed by symptoms of thyroid dysfunction should be suspected of having pituitary failure.

**361. The answer is B.** *(Speroff, ed 2. pp 118, 128-132, 236-240, 242.)* Because the woman described in the question is able to menstruate, she clearly does not have either Turner's or Reifenstein's syndrome. Kallman's syndrome is hypogonadotropic amenorrhea; women who have this disease rarely have increased androgen-production rates. The differential diagnosis in the case rests then between Stein-Leventhal syndrome and the adrenogenital syndrome. Women who have adrenogenital syndrome are virilized and have a muscular physique, an enlarged clitoris, and temporal recession of hair. That this patient shows only hirsutism indicates that the diagnosis is Stein-Leventhal syndrome.

**362. The answer is C.** *(Yen, pp 368, 451.)* Postpill amenorrhea affects fewer than 1 percent of women who have taken oral contraceptives. Because many women among this 1 percent relate a history of prior hypothalamic-pituitary dysfunction, it is important to distinguish postpill amenorrhea from amenor-

## Menstrual and Endocrine Disorders 165

rhea caused by endometrial involution. Although most cases of postpill amenorrhea resolve spontaneously within a few months, ovulation-inducing drugs such as clomiphene may be used provided that any serious underlying pathology is ruled out before the initiation of treatment.

**363. The answer is C (2, 4).** *(Green, ed 3. p 156.)* Recurring catamenial pneumothorax is a disorder of regularly ovulating women and can be prevented by therapy aimed at the suppression of ovulation. It only occurs during menses and is apparently due to alveolar rupture caused by an as-yet-unidentified sequela of normal ovulation. Examination of an affected lung shows little, if any, underlying pathology. In contrast to cyclic hemoptysis, recurring catamenial pneumothorax is not associated with endometriosis. The phenomenon is limited to the right thorax.

**364. The answer is E (all).** *(Rutledge, pp 108-109.)* Endometrial hyperplasia tends to develop in those women who also are at significant risk for developing adenocarcinoma of the endometrium. Hyperplasia is associated with unopposed estrogen stimulation of the endometrium, which occurs most often as a woman approaches menopause. However, it also may be associated with prolonged anovulation (as seen occasionally in postpartum women), with Stein-Leventhal syndrome, and with functioning ovarian tumors, such as granulosa-theca-cell tumor.

**365. The answer is B (1, 3).** *(Speroff, ed 2. p 107.)* Asherman's syndrome is intrauterine synechia that usually follows a too-vigorous postpartum curettage. Affected women continue to ovulate, although they do not have menstrual bleeding; their basic body temperatures, therefore, are biphasic and normal. The diagnosis of Asherman's syndrome is made by hysteroscopy or by hysterosalpingography. The etiology is not related to insertion of an intrauterine device (IUD), but IUDs have been utilized in treatment, because they separate the walls of the uterus after the adhesions are broken. However, a pediatric Foley catheter appears to be a better method of effecting the separation. After placement of the catheter, affected women should begin taking high doses of estrogen for 3 weeks a month, allowing the endometrium to regenerate.

**366. The answer is A (1, 2, 3).** *(Speroff, ed 2. p 151.)* Estrogen withdrawal bleeding, estrogen breakthrough bleeding, and progesterone breakthrough bleeding are mechanisms of dysfunctional uterine bleeding, which is defined as bleeding that does not occur according to a normal cycle. Progesterone withdrawal bleeding is the mechanism by which normal menstrual flow commences. A woman normally ovulates on day 14, and the corpus luteum begins producing progesterone. When progesterone production ceases about 14 days later, menstruation ensues.

**367. The answer is B (1, 3).** *(Isselbacher, ed 9. pp 416-420. Williams, ed 5. p 58.)* Patients who have anorexia nervosa, a loss of appetite due to emotional reasons, show a striking loss of body mass on physical examination; patients who have panhypopituitarism, however, show marked wasting only infrequently. Axillary and pubic hair are not lost in patients affected by anorexia nervosa, because circulating steroid levels are maintained. Steroid levels in panhypopituitarism, on the other hand, are low, causing loss of axillary and pubic hair. In panhypopituitarism, the human growth hormone level is extremely low and thyroid activity is decreased significantly; these values are either normal or elevated in anorectic individuals.

**368. The answer is A (1, 2, 3).** *(Williams, ed 5. pp 449-459, 484-487.)* The degree of mammary-gland development depends on the relationship between estrogen and androgen production and utilization. Development of mammary tissue is significant in individuals who have testicular feminization, in which peripheral testosterone use is very low; Refenstein's syndrome, in which serum testosterone levels are reduced; or Klinefelter's syndrome, in which testosterone production is decreased but estrogen production remains normal or near normal. On the other hand, mammary-gland development is not characteristic of Turner's syndrome patients, who produce no androgen and very little estrogen.

**369. The answer is E (all).** *(Williams, ed 5. p 56.)* Postpartum panhypopituitarism is caused by hemorrhage in and subsequent necrosis of the pituitary gland, which is enlarged during pregnancy. Temporal arteritis and sickle cell anemia lead to panhypopituitarism by causing chronic vascular insufficiency of the pituitary gland. Hand-Schüller-Christian disease causes panhypopituitarism as a result of the infiltration of the gland by cholesterol-laden histiocytes. In the empty-sella syndrome, the pituitary gland becomes compressed within the sella. The pressure eventually necroses the tissue, and the gland becomes nonfunctional.

**370. The answer is A (1, 2, 3).** *(Speroff, ed 2. pp 97-102.)* In the workup of primary amenorrhea, serum FSH and LH determinations can help to establish whether a woman has primary pituitary failure. A karyotype is important to rule out a genetic etiology, such as Turner's syndrome. Determination of serum prolactin levels is now practicable and becoming more popular in the workup of amenorrhea. (Prolactin is elevated in many of the pituitary microadenomas causing amenorrhea.) An endometrial biopsy in the workup of primary amenorrhea is of no value whatsoever.

**371. The answer is A (1, 2, 3).** *(Speroff, ed 2. pp 104-106.)* The CAT scan that accompanies the question depicts a coronal section of the skull; the midline

Menstrual and Endocrine Disorders 167

spherical area represents the sella turcica. In this study, the sella turcica is perfectly symmetric and normal in size. In the empty-sella syndrome, the sella is basically normal in configuration; a portion of arachnoid membrane herniates down through the diaphragm and compresses the active pituitary gland. Because microadenomas of the pituitary gland, which can produce prolactin and thus cause amenorrhea and galactorrhea, are usually less than 5 mm in size, they would not appear in the CAT scan shown. A suprasellar lesion of the pituitary gland would be larger than 5 mm and therefore would appear on most CAT scans.

**372. The answer is A (1, 2, 3).** *(Yen, pp 347-348.)* Anorexia nervosa is characterized by self-induced starvation and emaciation in the absence of organic disease. It is seen most commonly in adolescent girls and rarely occurs in boys. Most affected individuals have an obsessive-compulsive personality. It has been shown that the mean 24-hour cortisol concentration is twice normal because of increased circulation half-life and a decreased metabolic clearance rate. The daily cortisol production remains unchanged. These patients also have a low triiodothyronine ($T_3$) syndrome; both $T_3$ and thyroxine ($T_4$) are below normal values, with $T_3$ at a much lower level probably due to a disturbance in the peripheral conversion of $T_4$ to $T_3$.

**373. The answer is B (1, 3).** *(Speroff, ed 2. p 116. Yen, p 366.)* The empty-sella syndrome is a well-known condition in which an extension of the subarachnoid space is formed by the sella turcica. Pneumoencephalography, which will fill this space with air, is used as a diagnostic tool. Sella turcica x-ray usually reveals symmetrical enlargements. Individuals affected by this syndrome are frequently middle-aged women who are obese. The symptoms are generally nonspecific, with headaches being the most common complaint. The empty-sella syndrome is a benign condition that does not lead to pituitary failure. Inadvertent treatment for a pituitary tumor is probably the greatest hazard to the patient.

**374. The answer is E (all).** *(Romney, ed 2. pp 889-890.)* Primary dysmenorrhea is painful menstruation in the absence of pelvic disease that generally begins with the onset of regular ovulatory cycles. It is characterized by a combination of physical symptoms, such as pelvic cramps, nausea, vomiting, headache, and dizziness; and psychological symptoms, such as irritability, tension, and depression. Physical examination, including pelvic examination, is generally entirely normal. Recent investigations suggest that the symptomatology is caused by the local and systemic effects of prostaglandins released from menstrual fluid. Some investigators have reported an incidence of severe dysmenorrhea in 12 percent of women and moderate to severe dysmenorrhea in 45 percent of women. This frequency decreases with increasing parity.

**375-378. The answers are: 375-C, 376-D, 377-B, 378-A.** *(Speroff, ed 2. pp 158-159.)* The four women described in the question represent the four different patterns of menstrual bleeding. The first woman is not ovulating, and because she is producing estrogen (in varying amounts) she continues to stimulate her endometrium; the endometrium grows to a point where it sloughs. This woman's bleeding thus is called estrogen breakthrough bleeding.

The second woman has estrogen withdrawal bleeding. She is producing very little estrogen or progesterone. Exogenous estrogen stimulates her endometrium to grow, but as soon as this stimulus is taken away the endometrium no longer has nutritive support and therefore is sloughed.

The third woman, who demonstrates progesterone withdrawal bleeding, represents a normally ovulating woman. At the end of 14 days, the corpus luteum stops producing progesterone and the endometrium loses its structural support and therefore is sloughed.

The fourth woman is taking birth-control pills and has a high progesterone-to-estrogen ratio. If the amount of progesterone is not high enough to support the endometrium in the early phases, and if structural support is poor, the endometrium will break down and the woman will have progesterone breakthrough bleeding.

**379-383. The answers are: 379-D, 380-B, 381-A, 382-A, 383-C.** *(Speroff, ed 2. p 71. Williams, ed 5. pp 395-398, 808-813.)* True sexual precocity in girls is characterized by elevated gonadotropin levels and a normal ovulatory pattern. It represents premature activation of a normally operating hypothalamus-pituitary relationship. Although it usually is idiopathic, true sexual precocity can arise from cerebral causes as well as from hypothyroidism, polyostotic fibrous dysplasia, neurofibromatosis, and other disorders.

In girls who have precocious pseudopuberty, the endocrine glands, usually under neoplastic influences, produce elevated amounts of estrogens (isosexual precocious pseudopuberty) or androgens (heterosexual precocious pseudopuberty). Ovarian tumors appear to be the most common cause of isosexual precocious pseudopuberty; and some ovarian tumors, including dysgerminomas and choriocarcinomas, can produce so much gonadotropin that pregnancy tests are positive.

Incomplete sexual precocity, which usually is idiopathic, is characterized by only partial sexual maturity, such as premature thelarche, premature pubarche, or premature adrenarche. Incomplete sexual precocity can be accompanied by abnormal central-nervous-system function (e.g., mental deficiency).

In gonadotropin-producing tumors, high levels of gonadotropins, such as FSH, are produced with subsequent production of estrogen. Examples of these tumors are hepatoma, chorioepithelioma, and presacral tumors.

# Pelvic Relaxation, Infections, Endometriosis, and Infertility

**DIRECTIONS**: Each question below contains five suggested answers. Choose the **one best** response to each question.

384. An enterocele is best characterized by which of the following statements?

(A) It is not a true hernia
(B) It is a herniation of the bladder floor into the vagina
(C) It is a prolapse of the uterus and vaginal wall outside the body
(D) It is a protrusion of the pelvic peritoneal sac and vaginal wall into the vagina
(E) It is a herniation of the rectal and vaginal wall into the vagina

385. A 22-year-old woman comes to your office for a labial sore that she first noticed 2 days ago. Physical examination reveals a small ulcer of the right labium majus. Until other information is available, which of the following disorders should be considered the primary diagnosis?

(A) Chancroid
(B) Primary syphilis
(C) Lymphogranuloma inguinale
(D) Herpes simplex infection
(E) Early carcinoma of the vulva

386. All of the following steps are appropriate in the management of a woman who has a ruptured tubo-ovarian abscess EXCEPT

(A) preoperative antibiotic coverage consisting of penicillin and an aminoglycoside
(B) preoperative blood transfusions
(C) rapidly performed surgery (subtotal hysterectomy)
(D) bilateral salpingo-oophorectomy
(E) constant postoperative intestinal suction

387. All of the following statements about herpes genitalis are true EXCEPT that

(A) affected women may present with urinary retention
(B) many affected women have accompanying trichomoniasis or *Hemophilus vaginalis* vaginitis
(C) primary infections can be asymptomatic
(D) recurrent lesions tend to be disseminated and conspicuous
(E) use of tricyclic dyes can shorten the clinical course

388. Which of the following statements about pelvic tuberculosis is true?

(A) The primary site of involvement is the endometrium
(B) Infertility is a late complication
(C) The diagnosis can be made by endometrial biopsy
(D) The PPD skin test is positive in about half of affected women
(E) Treatment often restores fertility

389. Postpartum or postabortal pelvic inflammatory disease differs from gonorrheal pelvic inflammatory disease in all of the following respects EXCEPT

(A) the invasive quality of the organisms involved
(B) the vulnerability of the tissue to vascular spread
(C) the relative incidence of generalized sepsis
(D) the manifestations of the chronic phase of infection
(E) the potential for mortality

390. An 18-year-old woman comes to the emergency room with a complaint of vague lower abdominal pain for 1 week. Vital signs are stable except for a temperature of 37.8°C (100°F). Examination reveals tender adnexa bilaterally. Laparoscopy is performed and reveals bilateral hydrosalpinx. The next step in the management of this patient should be

(A) total abdominal hysterectomy and bilateral salpingectomy
(B) appropriate intravenous antibiotics
(C) bilateral salpingectomy
(D) posterior colpotomy
(E) further observation

391. A 17-year-old girl comes to your office complaining of a foul-smelling vaginal discharge that is causing her a great deal of discomfort. On performing a speculum examination, a foamy, yellowish discharge is seen in the posterior fornix, and multiple petechiae are seen in the cervix. The most likely pathogen is

(A) *Candida albicans*
(B) *Trichomonas vaginalis*
(C) *Hemophilus vaginalis*
(D) *Hemophilus ducreyi*
(E) β-hemolytic streptococci

392. A 39-year-old woman (gravida 2, para 2), who complains of pelvic pain, is found on laparoscopy to have extensive endometriosis. She does not want more children. The most appropriate treatment would be

(A) danazol
(B) oral contraceptives
(C) radical hysterectomy (Wertheim's operation)
(D) total abdominal hysterectomy with conservation of uninvolved ovaries
(E) total abdominal hysterectomy and bilateral salpingo-oophorectomy

393. The most common site of endometriosis is the

(A) uterine surface
(B) anterior cul-de-sac
(C) uterosacral ligaments
(D) ovary
(E) rectovaginal septum

394. All of the following statements about endometriosis are true EXCEPT that

(A) malignant changes are rare
(B) a diagnosis is established by history and physical examination
(C) it is more common in women in their reproductive years than in postmenopausal women
(D) affected women may present with infertility
(E) the most common site of involvement is the ovary

395. The photomicrograph below shows a portion of uterine wall from a 43-year-old woman who has chronic pelvic pain and dysmenorrhea that is unresponsive to hormonal therapy. The most likely diagnosis is

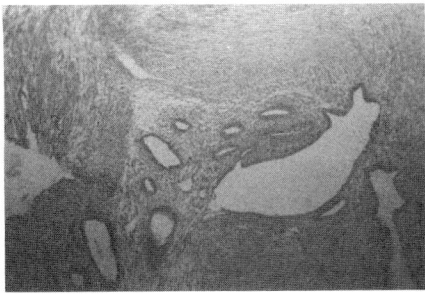

(A) endometriosis
(B) adenomyosis
(C) endometrial carcinoma
(D) ovarian carcinoma
(E) squamous cell carcinoma of the vulva

396. A 25-year-old woman comes to your office complaining of dyspareunia and intermittent, vague, lower abdominal pain unrelieved by analgesics. Pelvic examination reveals the presence of a thickened, nodular, right uterosacral ligament, and on laparoscopy, several "powder-burn" spots are seen in the pelvis. Initial treatment should consist of

(A) laparotomy with excision of the lesions
(B) total abdominal hysterectomy with bilateral salpingo-oophorectomy
(C) combination contraceptive pills on a continuous basis
(D) radiation therapy
(E) combination contraceptive pills on a cyclic basis

397. Which is the most common sign of impending evisceration from a wound incision?

(A) Serous drainage
(B) Sanguineous drainage
(C) Serosanguineous drainage
(D) Abdominal pain with no drainage
(E) Abdominal contents in the wound

398. Right ovarian vein syndrome is often associated with all of the following EXCEPT

(A) recurring right flank pain
(B) repeated episodes of right pyelonephritis
(C) cyclic hematuria
(D) premenstrual venous congestion
(E) appearance in women who have been pregnant at least once

399. A woman has been anuric for the first 48 hours after undergoing abdominal hysterectomy. Bilateral ligation of the ureters is suspected. Which of the following therapeutic measures should first be ordered?

(A) Observation only
(B) Ureteral catheterization
(C) Rapid dialysis
(D) Transabdominal deligation
(E) Bilateral nephrostomy

400. An extremely anxious 50-year-old woman presents to your office and complains of soaking her underpants when arising in the morning. She also reveals that once initiated, she is unable to control micturition. The most likely diagnosis is

(A) detrusor dyssynergia
(B) short-urethra syndrome
(C) urgency incontinence
(D) urethral diverticulum
(E) overflow incontinence

DIRECTIONS: Each question below contains four suggested answers of which one or more is correct. Choose the answer:

| A | if | 1, 2, and 3 | are correct |
|---|---|---|---|
| B | if | 1 and 3 | are correct |
| C | if | 2 and 4 | are correct |
| D | if | 4 | is correct |
| E | if | 1, 2, 3, and 4 | are correct |

401. A 27-year-old woman has an increased vaginal discharge, lower abdominal pain, and a low-grade fever; a neisserial infection is suspected. Appropriate culture media for the identification of *Neisseria gonorrhoeae* from the cervix include

(1) thioglycollate broth
(2) blood agar in a candle jar
(3) blood agar in an anaerobic chamber
(4) Thayer-Martin medium in a candle jar

402. Which of the following conditions can predispose to vaginal infection with *Candida albicans*?

(1) Pregnancy
(2) Antibiotic therapy
(3) Adrenocorticosteroid therapy
(4) Presence of an intrauterine device

403. Chancroid (soft chancre) can be characterized by which of the following statements?

(1) It is often accompanied by inguinal lymphadenopathy
(2) Diagnosis can be made by a complement fixation test
(3) Ducrey's bacillus (*Hemophilus ducreyi*) is the causative agent
(4) Affected individuals are best treated with a course of tetracycline

404. Treatments commonly employed for women who have the vulvar lesion shown below include

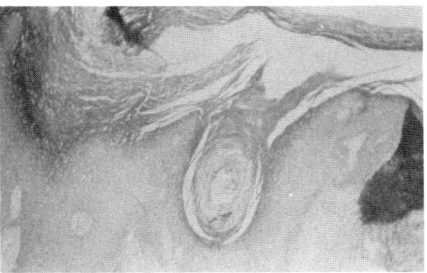

(1) podophyllum
(2) 5-fluorouracil
(3) cryosurgery
(4) simple vulvectomy

405. Histological features that are diagnostic for endometriosis include

(1) endometrial glands
(2) evidence of hemorrhage
(3) endometrial stroma
(4) decidual reaction in the surrounding tissue

406. The symptoms of endometriosis can include

(1) pain during defecation
(2) abnormal uterine bleeding
(3) dyspareunia
(4) progressive primary dysmenorrhea

## SUMMARY OF DIRECTIONS

| A | B | C | D | E |
|---|---|---|---|---|
| 1, 2, 3 only | 1, 3 only | 2, 4 only | 4 only | All are correct |

407. At the present time, treatment of women who have endometriosis can consist of single-agent therapy with
(1) androgens
(2) progestational agents
(3) nonsteroidal gonadotropin inhibitors
(4) estrogens

408. Retrograde menstruation is the most accepted explanation of the etiology of endometriosis. Which of the following statements may be cited as evidence for this theory?
(1) Inversion of the cervix of a monkey into the peritoneal cavity can cause endometriosis
(2) Endometrial tissue can be cultured successfully
(3) Menstrual blood can come from the ends of the fallopian tubes of some women
(4) Endometrial glands can arise from coelomic epithelium

409. Luteal-phase defect is associated with faulty ovulation. Which of the following studies performed in the second half of the menstrual cycle would be helpful in making a diagnosis?
(1) Serum progesterone levels
(2) Urine pregnanetriol levels
(3) Endometrial biopsy
(4) Serum luteinizing hormone levels

410. During gynecological surgery, operative injuries to the ureter occur
(1) more frequently in association with vaginal rather than abdominal hysterectomy
(2) only rarely if periureteral tissue is dissected carefully
(3) most commonly when the ureter lies between the anterior vaginal wall and the base of the bladder
(4) often as a result of hasty reclamping of vessel clamps or ligatures

411. The x-ray shown below reveals which of the following?

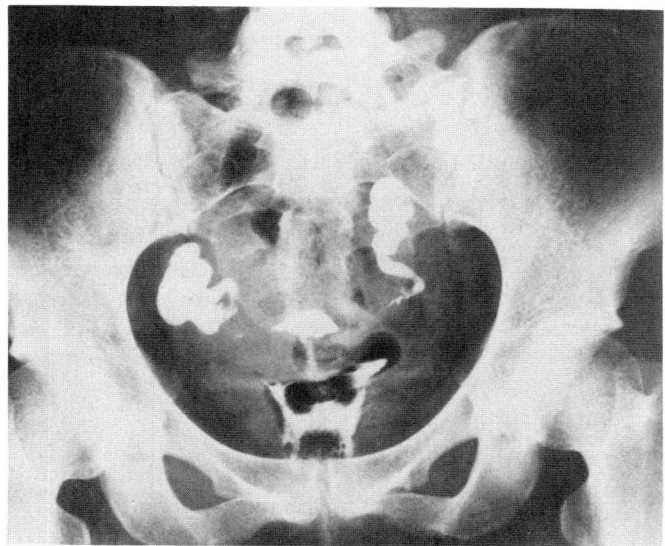

(1) Cornual obstruction
(2) Distended tubes
(3) Bilateral spill
(4) Bilateral hydrosalpinx

412. If ureteral injury is recognized at the time of surgery, which of the following procedures could be recommended?

(1) A longitudinal slit should be made in the ureter below the injury and a polyethylene tube threaded into the bladder
(2) If the ureter is not severed, the site of injury should be drained intraperitoneally
(3) If the ureter is severed, uretero-ureteral anastomosis should be attempted, regardless of the location of the injury
(4) If possible, the severed ureter should be implanted into the bladder

413. Lymphogranuloma venereum, the incidence of which has been increasing in the United States, can be described by which of the following statements?

(1) It usually is accompanied by unilateral inguinal adenitis
(2) It can involve the anus, rectum, and sigmoid colon
(3) Affected women usually are unresponsive to penicillin
(4) Diagnosis by the Frei test is common

DIRECTIONS: The groups of questions below consist of lettered choices followed by several numbered items. For each numbered item select the **one** lettered choice with which it is **most** closely associated. Each lettered choice may be used once, more than once, or not at all.

## Questions 414-417

For each description that follows, select the operative procedure with which it is most likely to be associated.

(A) Salpingoplasty
(B) Salpingostomy
(C) Salpingolysis
(D) Fimbriolysis
(E) Uterotubal implantation

414. Forming a patent entry site in the fundal portion of the uterus and attaching the oviduct

415. Section of adhesions causing conglutination of the distal end of the oviduct

416. Cutting adhesions around the uterine tube

417. Opening up a previously formed hydrosalpinx

## Questions 418-422

Match the following.

(A) *Candida albicans*
(B) *Trichomonas vaginalis*
(C) *Neisseria gonorrhoeae*
(D) *Corynebacterium vaginale* (*Hemophilus vaginalis*)
(E) Atrophic (senile) vaginitis

418. A frequent cause of nonspecific vaginitis

419. Diabetes mellitus may be a predisposing factor

420. Typically produces a frothy discharge

421. Typically produces a grossly recognizable, punctate hemorrhagic vaginal mucosa ("strawberry spots")

422. Treatment with an estrogen cream may be effective

## Questions 423-427

For each clinical description that follows, select the appropriate disorder.

(A) Neurogenic bladder
(B) Overflow incontinence
(C) Stress incontinence
(D) Vesicovaginal fistula
(E) Urgency incontinence

423. A 45-year-old woman states that she has had increasing difficulty holding urine after feeling the need to void. She occasionally loses urine when sitting down

424. A 43-year-old woman, who recently underwent an anterior vaginal repair, complains of constant perineal wetness and loss of urine while standing. She does not feel the urge to void

425. A 28-year-old diabetic woman reports that she loses large volumes of urine without warning. She says that she can overcome the problem by frequent, voluntary emptying of the bladder

426. A 26-year-old woman, who has four children, is worried because her daily jogging seems to be causing urinary dribbling

427. An 83-year-old woman, who lives in a nursing home, complains that dribbling of urine, which had occurred only when she was walking, now is markedly aggravated by a cold

## Questions 428-431

For each clinical presentation that follows, select the antibiotic with which it should be treated.

(A) Gentamicin
(B) Ampicillin
(C) Tetracycline
(D) Cephalothin
(E) A sulfonamide antibiotic

428. A 23-year-old woman who has had a septic abortion has positive blood cultures with an organism that is identified as an aerobic gram-negative rod

429. A 28-year-old woman who is in her thirty-seventh week of pregnancy develops a urinary tract infection with *Escherichia coli*

430. A 34-year-old single woman develops a *Mycoplasma hominis* infection

431. A 28-year-old woman at 4 weeks gestation develops asymptomatic bacteriuria

## Questions 432-435

A 48-year-old woman enters the hospital for a total abdominal hysterectomy and bilateral salpingo-oophorectomy, which is performed on the first hospital day. The woman's temperatures, recorded for her first 8 days of hospitalization, are shown below. Realizing that postoperative pyrexia can stem from many causes, match the postoperative day with the therapeutic measure below that is most likely to be instituted during that day.

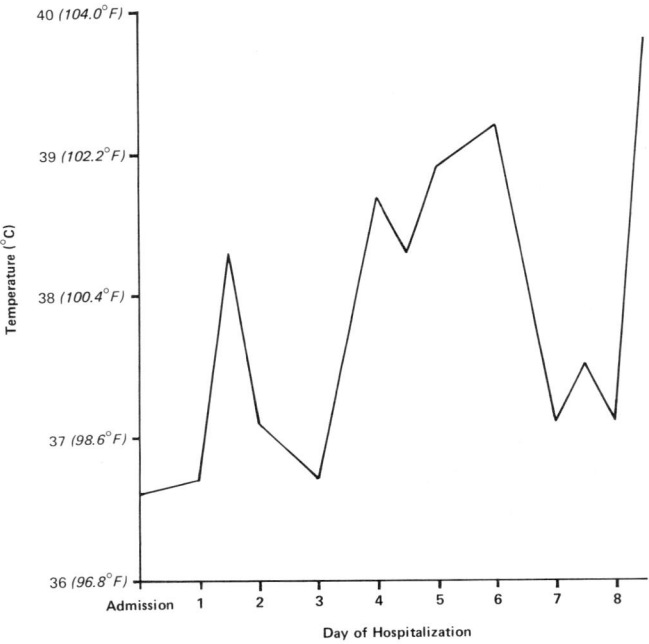

(A) Administration of heparin
(B) Administration of ampicillin
(C) Administration of chloramphenicol or clindamycin
(D) Intermittent positive-pressure breathing and deep-breathing exercises
(E) Vaginal or abdominal drainage

432. Day one (first night after surgery)

433. Day four

434. Day five

435. Day six

# Pelvic Relaxation, Infections, Endometriosis, and Infertility

# Answers

**384. The answer is D.** *(Mattingly, ed 5. pp 603-607.)* An enterocele is the protrusion of the pelvic peritoneal sac and the vaginal wall into the vagina. It is a true hernia, and it may be either congenital or associated with a uterine prolapse. Enteroceles can also occur following vaginal hysterectomy if the cul-de-sac is not adequately obliterated. Most commonly, patients with enteroceles complain of a mass protruding from the vagina when they strain, cough, sneeze, or perform other activities associated with the Valsalva maneuver—that is, activities causing pressure (by exhalation) against a closed glottis. Also, if intestines are present in the herniated sac, local discomfort will probably result.

**385. The answer is B.** *(Kistner, ed 3. pp 31-32.)* The gross appearance of genital ulcers may give little information about the underlying disease process. Primary syphilis, chancroid, herpes simplex, lymphogranuloma inguinale, and early vulvar carcinoma all may be associated wtih ulcerative lesions; in addition, the "classic" hard ulcer of syphilis may, in fact, be soft, and the soft lesion of chancroid, hard. Experience has shown that, until ruled out, syphilis must be considered the primary diagnosis.

**386. The answer is A.** *(Mattingly, ed 5. pp 268-271.)* An important aspect that is often overlooked in the management of a woman who has a tubo-ovarian abscess is preoperative antibiotic coverage for *Bacteroides fragilis*. Because penicillin combined with an aminoglycoside can cover all potential pathogens except *B. fragilis*, clindamycin, carbenicillin, or chloramphenicol should be added to the antibiotic regimen. Because patients are put in Trendelenberg position, rapid surgery is required; thus, a subtotal hysterectomy frequently is performed. For most patients, bilateral salpingo-oophorectomy also is indicated, and postoperative intestinal suction is recommended.

**387. The answer is D.** *(Romney, ed 2. pp 924-925.)* The symptoms of primary herpes genitalis, which include blisters, ulcers, pain, and urinary retention, are often severe and may persist for several weeks. Several studies have shown that a number of women who show no signs of herpes genitalis have antibodies to herpes simplex virus type 2, the causative agent of the disease; this finding indicates that these women have had previous, asymptomatic infections. Recurrent infections, which occur commonly, are localized and often hard to identify. At present, herpetic lesions are treated symptomatically with local application of topical anesthetics and antibiotics in conjunction with sitz baths. Other modes of therapy, such as photoinactivation with tricyclic dyes, 5-IUDR (idoxuridine), and Ara-A, have not been proven to be effective or safe.

**388. The answer is C.** *(Green, ed 3. pp 270-272. Willson, ed 6. pp 545-546.)* Pelvic tuberculosis is usually secondary to tuberculous infection in another part of the body—most often the lung. It is thought that the infection spreads hematogenously from the fallopian tubes—the primary site of pelvic infection—into the endometrial cavity. Although the endometrium is only secondarily affected, endometrial biopsy often is the easiest method of diagnosis. The tuberculin skin (PPD) test usually is positive. Affected women most often present with pelvic pain, dysmenorrhea, dyspareunia, irregular menses, and cervical lesions. In view of primary tubal involvement, infertility is an early manifestation; and even with proper treatment, affected women have only a poor chance of regaining their childbearing capacity.

**389. The answer is D.** *(Green, ed 3. pp 256-269.)* The pathogenesis and presentation of postabortal or postpartum pelvic inflammatory disease, which is extremely life-threatening, differ in a number of respects from gonorrheal pelvic inflammatory disease. The relatively unprotected vessels of the gravid uterus are easy portals for vascular entry of bacteria, which probably is a major reason for the increased incidence of generalized sepsis. The organisms responsible for these infections (gram-negative bacteria are the most common) are often more invasive and destructive than gonococci, which tend to spread superficially along the mucosa. In general, however, the manifestations of chronic infections and the management of affected women are similar.

**390. The answer is B.** *(Mattingly, ed 5. pp 259-264.)* In the initial mangement of an acute pelvic infection, the use of surgery is rarely indicated. Laparoscopy is a useful tool for providing a definitive diagnosis and indicating the extent of the disease. In most cases of acute pelvic infection, 24 to 72 hours of appropriate intravenous antibiotic therapy followed by 1 week of oral therapy will produce a positive response. Definitive surgery can be recommended for the older patient whose childbearing functions have been fulfilled. Posterior colpotomy is performed for the purpose of establishing drainage, when the abscess is fluctuant and located in the midline.

**391. The answer is B.** *(Green, ed 3. p 277. Parsons, ed 2. pp 766, 771.)* Foamy, foul discharge accompanied by cervical petechiae, which are often described as "strawberrylike" in appearance, confirms the diagnosis of trichomoniasis. The latter finding is not seen in any other form of vaginitis. In candidiasis, the discharge is less abundant, and on speculum examination, thick, cheeselike plaques can be seen clinging to the vaginal mucosa. Infection with *Hemophilus vaginalis* produces a grayish, malodorous discharge and does not cause as much intense itching and burning as the previous two pathogens described. *Hemophilus ducreyi* is the causative organism of chancroid (soft chancre).

**392. The answer is E.** *(Speroff, ed 2. pp 356-360.)* Because the woman described in the question does not want more children, the definitive and only curative procedure would be a total abdominal hysterectomy and bilateral salpingo-oophorectomy. Retaining any ovarian tissue would be contraindicated, because the constant production of hormone would stimulate the endometrial implants not detected during the original surgery and thus would cause the patient's symptoms to recur. The use of danazol, an antigonadotropin, or oral contraceptives to treat the woman described would only suppress and decidualize the endometrial implants. Both treatments are temporary measures only.

**393. The answer is D.** *(Mattingly, ed 5. pp 228-233. Romney, ed 2. p 933.)* The most common site of endometriosis is the ovary. Superficial serosal lesions also are common, especially on the uterine and tubal surfaces and in scattered locations on the pelvic serosa. Endometrial implants may also be found on the uterosacral ligaments, round ligaments, in the rectovaginal septum, on the pelvic peritoneum covering the uterus, tubes, rectum, sigmoid, or bladder, at the umbilicus, in laparotomy scars, hernial sacs, the appendix, vagina, vulva, cervix, tubal stumps, or lymph nodes.

**394. The answer is B.** *(Romney, ed 2. pp 932-933, 938-940.)* Endometriosis, which most commonly involves the ovaries, is a disease of women in their reproductive years, especially between the ages of 30 and 40 years. The disease is usually benign. The definitive diagnosis of endometriosis rarely can be established short of surgery or diagnostic laparoscopy. Diagnosis is aided by the presence of vulvar, vaginal, or cervical lesions, which can be biopsied; palpable cul-de-sac nodules; and a history of dysmenorrhea and infertility.

**395. The answer is B.** *(Novak, ed 8. pp 280-290.)* The histological and historical evidence presented in the question suggests adenomyosis. Adenomyosis is defined as endometrial tissue outside of the endometrial cavity and confined to the uterine wall. Tufts of endometrial tissue can be surrounded by areas of smooth muscle (myometrium), as in the accompanying photomicrograph. Endometriosis is defined as endometrial tissue outside of the uterus. Because the lesion shown is certainly benign, ovarian carcinoma and carcinoma of the vulva are ruled out. Women who have adenomyosis suffer from chronic pelvic pain and dysmenorrhea, usually associated with an enlarged uterus. A diagnosis is rarely made clinically and usually depends on pathological examination.

**396. The answer is C.** *(Green, ed 3. pp 341-348.)* In situations where there are only minimal lesions of endometriosis in the cul-de-sac and along the uterosacral ligaments, noncyclic hormonal therapy in the form of combination oral contraceptives are used for 6 to 12 months. Endometriosis in young women can involve the adnexa in the form of dense adhesions or large endometriomas. In these cases conservative surgery that encompasses the removal of as much disease as possible and the preservation of as much of the organs necessary for reproduction as possible is recommended. Radiation therapy was the mode of therapy used in the past for ablation of the ovaries, which cut off the stimulus for the endometriotic lesions. Primarily because of the fear of possible later malignancy arising as a result of radiation, this form of treatment is not presently used for endometriosis.

**397. The answer is C.** *(Mattingly, ed 5. pp 176-179.)* Serosanguineous drainage occurs very frequently before evisceration from an incision. Drainage can be accompanied by pain or by the feeling that something is "giving way." Serous or sanguineous drainage often is noted postoperatively and usually suggests involvement of the superficial wound.

**398. The answer is C.** *(Green, ed 3. p 171.)* Right ovarian vein syndrome is a type of acquired menstrual pain. It usually appears in women who have been pregnant at least once. The cause is believed to be related to incompetence of the valves of the right ovarian vein that can result during pregnancy. The clinical course features recurring ureteral obstruction and subsequent recurring right flank pain and pyelonephritis; these symptoms are due to premenstrual venous pelvic congestion and enlargement of the right ovarian vein.

**399. The answer is B.** *(Mattingly, ed 5. pp 299-300.)* Bilateral ureteral obstruction, if unrecognized or unrelieved, can cause death in 7 to 10 days. Once the presence of bilateral ureteral obstruction is suspected, bilateral ureteral catheters should be passed in order to demonstrate and, if possible, overcome the obstructions. If obstruction persists, bilateral nephrostomy should be performed; if, 6 to 8 weeks later, the obstructions still cannot be overcome, ureteral surgery should be undertaken.

**400. The answer is A.** *(Green, ed 3. pp 552-556.)* True urinary stress incontinence results from a deficiency of the normal anatomical support of the bladder neck and urethra. The condition that most often mimics true urinary stress incontinence is detrusor dyssynergia, which in the majority of cases has a psychosomatic origin and often produces a "voiding" type of leakage associated with a change in position, such as arising from bed in the morning. The short-urethra syndrome results in continuous leakage of urine regardless of position or stress, and pure urgency incontinence, which is often secondary to a nonbacterial trigonitis or cystitis, often results in sudden, uncontrollable micturition. Urethral diverticula are not associated with incontinence. Overflow incontinence would be suggested by frequent voiding of **small** amounts of urine with a significant residual urine volume noted on catheterization.

**401. The answer is D (4).** *(Monif, pp 390-391.)* Selective media must be used for the identification of *Neisseria gonorrhoeae* taken from the genital tract. Cultures using nonselective media are likely to be overgrown with other pelvic bacteria. Culturing multiple sites, especially the anus and oropharynx, in addition to the cervix, can result in the detection of approximately 90 percent of gonorrheal infections in women; multiple-site culturing is best used as a means of monitoring the effectiveness of treatment.

**402. The answer is A (1, 2, 3).** *(Monif, pp 242-243.)* Pregnancy is associated with an increase in the incidence of monilial infections, probably because of an increase in glycogen content in the vaginal mucosa. Antibiotic therapy clearly increases the likelihood of candidiasis (moniliasis), perhaps because it eliminates susceptible bacteria that compete with *Candida* for available nutrients. Steroid therapy also increases the likelihood of candidiasis; the mechanism of action may involve inhibition of catabolic-enzyme release. No association exists between the use of intrauterine devices and a predisposition toward monilial infections.

**403. The answer is B (1, 3).** *(Green, ed 3. p 277. Romney, ed 2. pp 923-924.)* Chancroid (soft chancre) is a very contagious venereal disease that is caused by Ducrey's bacillus (*Hemophilus ducreyi*). Painful, tender lesions of the external genitalia usually appear 3 to 10 days after a sexual encounter with an infected individual. Development of these lesions frequently is followed by enlargement of inguinal lymph nodes. Diagnosis is usually made by a culture of the ulcerated lesion; and treatment of affected individuals is with a 2-week course of tetracycline (250 mg four times a day) or sulfadazine (1 g four times a day).

**404. The answer is B (1, 3).** *(Novak, ed 8. pp 28-30.)* The lesion shown in the figure accompanying the question is condyloma acuminatum, also known as a venereal wart; it is a squamous lesion caused by the papilloma virus. The lesion reveals a treelike growth microscopically, with a mantle that shows marked acanthosis and parakeratosis. Occasionally hyperkeratosis is noted. The treatment is local excision, cryosurgery, or podophyllum, which is a locally acting, mild antimetabolite. 5-Fluorouracil is a very potent antimetabolite, and simple vulvectomy is too expensive and radical a surgical procedure for removal of this benign, self-limiting lesion.

**405. The answer is A (1, 2, 3).** *(Green, ed 3. p 334.)* In view of the importance of accuracy in diagnosing endometriosis, strict, definitive criteria must be used. The triad of histological findings that is diagnostic for endometriosis consists of the presence of endometrial glands and endometrial stroma and evidence of recent or old hemorrhage. In women who are pregnant or who are receiving certain forms of hormonal therapy, a significant decidual reaction may be seen; this feature, however, is by no means diagnostic for endometriosis.

**406. The answer is A (1, 2, 3).** *(Romney, ed 2. pp 938-939.)* The severity and frequency of the symptoms of endometriosis are variable. Pelvic pain, which may take the form of acquired dysmenorrhea, dyspareunia, or painful defecation, is the most common presenting complaint. Abnormal patterns of urinary bleeding probably result from local alterations due to ovarian involvement rather than from central hormonal dysfunction. In rare cases, the spontaneous rupture of endometrial cysts produce a medical emergency. Some patients present with infertility; however, it is unclear how endometriosis affects fertility.

**407. The answer is A (1, 2, 3).** *(Green, ed 3. pp 342-344.)* The major hormonal agents used at this time in the treatment of women who have endometriosis are progestins and androgens. Hormonal therapy has proved especially useful for women whose symptoms are mild. Because pregnancy can lessen the severity of endometriosis, estrogen therapy was tried as a possible treatment; the incidence of side effects and complications proved to be quite high, however, and estrogens now are used only for treatment of women with breakthrough-type bleeding. Gonadotropin inhibition is now possible without the use of steroid therapy.

**408. The answer is A (1, 2, 3).** *(Speroff, ed 2. p 355.)* Retrograde menstruation is currently believed to be a major cause of endometriosis. Supporting this belief are the following findings: inversion of the uterine cervix into the peritoneal cavity can cause a monkey to develop endometriosis; endometrial tissue is

Infections, Endometriosis, and Infertility 185

viable outside the uterus; and blood can issue from the ends of the fallopian tubes of some women during menstruation. The fact that endometrial implants can occur in the lung implies that lymphatic or vascular routes of spread of the disease also are possible. Another theory of the etiology of endometriosis entails the conversion of coelomic epithelium into glands resembling those of the endometrium.

**409. The answer is B (1, 3).** *(Behrman, ed 2. pp 308-314.)* A short luteal phase is defined as ovulation with poor production of progesterone in the second half of the cycle. Progesterone levels at that time of less than 7 ng/ml are diagnostic. Endometrial biopsy also is crucial to the diagnosis of this defect, because the endometrium will be out of phase with the time of cycle. For example, a biopsy taken on day 26 of the cycle will resemble endometrium of day 24 because of decreased progesterone stimulation. Pregnanetriol is a breakdown product of 17-hydroxyprogesterone, and levels are not helpful in diagnosing this condition. Determination of the level of pregnanediol, which is a metabolic product of progesterone excreted in the urine, is a helpful test. Serum luteinizing hormone levels have no correlation with the presence of a luteal-phase defect.

**410. The answer is D (4).** *(Mattingly, ed 5. pp 293-295.)* Operative injuries to the ureter are associated more commonly with abdominal hysterectomy than vaginal hysterectomy. The most common site of injury occurs near the region of the uterine vessels. Because the blood supply to the ureter arises from the periureteral tissue, dissection should be avoided; even careful dissection results in a significant percentage of ureteral injuries, and the incidence of fistula formation is increased if the blood supply is compromised. Slippage of vessels from clamps or ligatures can lead to ureteral injury if the vessels are reclamped hastily in an effort to stop the resultant bleeding.

**411. The answer is C (2, 4).** *(Kistner, ed 3. pp 290-295.)* The x-ray presented reveals bilateral hydrosalpinx and distended tubes; no spill is noted at the fimbriated extremity. These findings are suggestive of chronic pelvic inflammatory disease. Both cornual areas appear normal, and there is no spill into the peritoneal cavity.

**412. The answer is D (4).** *(Mattingly, ed 5. pp 300-306.)* Following injury to the ureter during surgery, a drain should be placed extraperitoneally. If a polyethylene catheter is inserted, it should be placed above the site of injury so that urine is drained before arrival at the site of injury. Ureteroureteral anastomosis should be done only if reimplantation into the bladder is not feasible. Implanting a severed ureter into the bladder is the procedure of choice.

**413. The answer is E (all).** *(Green, ed 3. pp 277-278. Romney, ed 2. p 233.)* The etiologic agent of lymphogranuloma venereum is a nonmotile obligate intracellular parasite probably derived from gram negative bacteria. It differs from viruses in its possession of both DNA or RNA (one or the other with viruses), it multiplies by binary fission, possesses ribosomes and can be inhibited by antimicrobial drugs. Therefore, treatment with sulfonamides, chlortetracycline, or chloramphenicol is usually effective in the early stages of the infection. The initial prodrome (including fever and malaise) is followed by unilateral inguinal adenitis, which progresses to bubo formation. Lymphatic spread can lead to involvement of the anus, rectum, or sigmoid. The Frei skin test usually can diagnose lymphogranuloma venereum. Although it is primarily a disease of women who live in warm climates, lymphogranuloma venereum is on the increase in the United States, in part due to the return of the infected soldiers from Vietnam and neighboring countries.

**414-417. The answers are: 414-E, 415-D, 416-C, 417-B.** *(Behrman, ed 2. pp 224-225.)* Salpingolysis, salpingoplasty, and uterotubal implantation are the major surgical techniques utilized by tubal surgeons. A salpingolysis is merely the cutting of adhesions surrounding the fallopian tube. Salpingoplasty, which is performed on the fimbriated end of the tube, is divided into two parts: fimbriolysis, which is a simple cutting of adhesions causing the fimbria to conglutinate in the midline, and salpingostomy, which is creation of an opening in tubes that were completely closed with hydrosalpinx, usually secondary to infection. On occasion, the tube is occluded at the cornual area, which must be excised, and a new opening into the uterus must be created; this procedure is uterotubal implantation. These procedures are commonly used to correct infertility problems related to lack of tubal patency or mobility interfering with ovum pickup/transport. Predisposing factors include endometriosis, pelvic inflammatory disease, appendicitis, and prior tubal ligation.

**418-422. The answers are: 418-D, 419-A, 420-B, 421-B, 422-E.** *(Sciarra, pp 5, 8-12.)* Many cases of nonspecific vaginitis are caused by *Corynebacterium vaginale*. These women usually complain of a characteristic malodorous, grayish vaginal discharge. On wet mounts, the diagnosis is made by visualizing the "clue cells," which are epithelial cells with large numbers of adherent coccobacilli. The recommended treatment is ampicillin, although vaginal sulfa creams are also effective.

Besides diabetes mellitus, other predisposing factors of candidiasis include pregnancy, the use of antibiotics, immunosuppressive medications, and possibly oral contraceptives. Affected individuals usually complain of severe pruritus and thick, cheeselike vaginal discharge. Wet mounts show characteristic yeast cells and hyphae. The primary mode of treatment is the vaginal application of an antifungal agent, such as nystatin.

*Trichomonas vaginalis* classically gives rise to a yellowish, frothy discharge, which is foul smelling and causes pruritus. The pathognomonic "strawberry spots," which consist of punctate hemorrhagic spots on the vaginal mucosa, can sometimes be seen. The diagnosis is made by observing the characteristic motile protozoan on wet mounts. The mainstay of treatment is oral metronidazole, either in a single dose of 2 g or 250 mg three times a day for 7 to 10 days. Metronidazole has a disulfiramlike effect, and women taking it should refrain from consumption of alcohol. Vaginal suppositories of clotrimazole, 100 mg once a day for 7 days, are also effective and are preferred by some because of carcinogenicity found in rodents treated with metronidazole.

Postmenopausal women who present with symptoms like itching, irritation secondary to dryness, and dyspareunia often have atrophic (senile) vaginitis. Due to the lack of estrogen, the vaginal mucosa becomes very thin and easily irritable. This condition responds well to either oral intake of estrogen or local application of estrogen creams.

The Bartholin's glands, endocervical glands, and fallopian tubes can all be infected by *Neisseria gonorrhoeae*, but an infection of the vaginal mucosa is uncommon.

**423-427. The answers are: 423-E, 424-D, 425-A, 426-C, 427-B.** *(Romney, ed 2. pp 958-962.)* Urgency incontinence resulting from hyperactivity of the detrusor muscle is associated with the loss of large amounts of urine just after a woman has had an urge to void. Sudden motions can trigger the urge.

Small fistulas can result from improperly performed surgery that has created an unnoticed entry into the bladder. Affected patients, when recumbent, will pool urine in the vagina.

Diabetes as well as neurological disorders can be associated with neurogenic bladder. Reflex emptying, which usually is spasmodic and not accompanied by a sensation of a full bladder, is characteristic of the disorder.

Characteristically, stress incontinence is the loss of urine caused by sudden increases in intra-abdominal pressure. The condition is uncommon in women who never have been pregnant.

Conditions that cause pressure on or constriction of the bladder neck can lead to an overdistended bladder. Overflow incontinence also occurs not infrequently among elderly patients.

**428-431. The answers are: 428-A, 429-B, 430-C, 431-E.** *(Ledger, Clin Obstet Gynecol 20:417-418, 1977. Monif, pp 9, 26, 159. Romney, ed 2. p 725. Willson, pp 37, 426.)* Gentamicin, an aminoglycoside similar to kanamycin and streptomycin, is not absorbed after oral administration. It is the drug of choice for women who have severe infections caused by gram-negative aerobes.

The penicillins are nontoxic for pregnant women. Ampicillin is used effectively for treating urinary tract infections and acute pyelonephritis. Ampicillin can cause a decrease in the urinary excretion of estriol in pregnancy. The exact reason for this is unclear.

Although *Mycoplasma hominis* commonly is found in the genital tract, its role in producing infections is unclear. Documented mycoplasmal infections are best treated with tetracycline, unless the affected woman is pregnant, as tetracycline deposition in fetuses can cause abnormal bone growth and permanent mottling of the teeth. Also, large doses of the drug may cause hepatic degeneration in the mother.

Pregnant women with asymptomatic bacteriuria can be treated effectively and safely with sulfonamides up until the last month of pregnancy—after which sulfonamides are contraindicated. In late pregnancy, this antibiotic crosses the placenta and competes with bilirubin for binding sites in the fetus, which can lead to hyperbilirubinemia and kernicterus in the neonate.

**432-435. The answers are: 432-D, 433-B, 434-C, 435-E.** *(Romney, ed 2. pp 1262-1266.)* The hospital course of the patient described in the question reflects many of the diagnostic situations that can face a clinician. A rapid rise in temperature in the early postoperative period often can be traced to atelectasis; pulmonary problems can be treated by using intermittent positive-pressure breathing and by getting the patient to cough and perform deep-breathing exercises. Early pelvic cellulitis, which is responsible for the rise on day four of the patient's temperature, should be treated initially with standard antibiotic therapy, including the use of such medications as ampicillin. Failure to respond in 24 to 48 hours should suggest the presence of an anaerobic infection; appropriate therapy with, for example, chloramphenicol or clindamycin, should then be instituted. Because *Bacteroides* infections are associated with a high incidence of pelvic abscess, failure of a patient to respond to appropriate antibiotic treatment should prompt a search for this condition. The patient's fever on day eight might indicate recollection of a pelvic abscess or pelvic thrombophlebitis, which also is often associated with anaerobic infections.

# Benign and Malignant Neoplasms

**DIRECTIONS**: Each question below contains five suggested answers. Choose the **one best** response to each question.

436. A 42-year-old multiparous woman comes to your office complaining of irregular menses and frequent urination. Her pregnancy test is negative. Ultrasonography and physical examination suggest the presence of a fibroid uterus (i.e., leiomyoma of the uterus) that is twice normal size. An examination performed 6 months earlier revealed a normal-size uterus. A hysterectomy would be recommended because

(A) a fibroid uterus leads to abnormal bleeding
(B) a fibroid the size of a 2-month pregnancy must be removed
(C) fibroids have a high malignant potential
(D) urinary frequency suggests severe pressure symptoms
(E) rapid appearance of fibroids warrants the procedure

437. A 43-year-old multiparous woman has a 4-year history of irregular menses and frequent urination. Physical examination reveals an irregular uterus that is two or three times normal size. As the woman's physician, you now would

(A) perform a dilatation and curettage
(B) order a pregnancy test
(C) order ultrasonography
(D) order intravenous pyelography
(E) schedule a hysterectomy

438. Carcinoma in situ of the cervix is characterized by all of the following EXCEPT

(A) involvement of the entire thickness of the squamous epithelium
(B) cells resembling those of invasive carcinoma
(C) evidence of stromal invasion
(D) complete loss of stratification
(E) occasional regression and disappearance

439. All of the following statements about Brenner tumors of the ovary are true EXCEPT that

(A) they generally are benign
(B) they are characterized microscopically by areas of epithelial cells surrounded by mesenchymal tissue
(C) their cells have a characteristic "coffee-bean" nucleus
(D) they tend to grow rather slowly
(E) they rarely are larger than 2 cm in diameter

440. Pelvic examination of a 19-year-old woman who complains of lower abdominal discomfort reveals a mobile, 6-cm mass in the anterior cul-de-sac. The most likely diagnosis is

(A) serous carcinoma
(B) urachal cyst
(C) benign cystic teratoma
(D) intraligamentous fibroid
(E) diverticular abscess

441. Ovarian neoplasms most commonly arise from

(A) coelomic epithelium
(B) nonspecific mesenchyme
(C) specialized gonadal stroma
(D) primitive germ cells
(E) none of the above

442. The ovarian cyst or tumor that is most common during infancy and childhood is

(A) dermoid cyst
(B) theca-lutein cyst
(C) giant follicle cyst
(D) granuloma cell tumor
(E) benign solid teratoma

443. A 48-year-old woman presents with a nontender fluctuant mass in her right vulva that causes some discomfort when walking and during coitus and that is consistent with a diagnosis of Bartholin's cyst. What is the most appropriate treatment?

(A) Marsupialization
(B) Antibiotics
(C) Surgical excision
(D) Incision and drainage
(E) No treatment necessary

444. Stage IIb carcinoma of the cervix is defined by

(A) involvement only of the cervix with early stromal invasion
(B) extension to the corpus uteri without parametrial involvement
(C) extension beyond the cervix (but not to the pelvic wall or the lower one-third of the vagina) without obvious parametrial involvement
(D) extension beyond the cervix (but not to the pelvic wall or the lower one-third of the vagina) with obvious parametrial involvement
(E) extension to the pelvic wall and involvement of the upper one-third of the vagina

445. The neoplasm most sensitive to appropriate chemotherapy is

(A) gestational trophoblastic disease
(B) ovarian dysgerminoma
(C) Burkitt's lymphoma
(D) endometrial carcinoma
(E) ovarian serous carcinoma

446. A 25-year-old woman complains of diarrhea and weight loss; her heart rate is 130 per minute. Head, neck, and chest x-rays, upper gastrointestinal series, small-bowel follow-through, and barium enema all are negative. An ovarian lesion, discovered during laparotomy, is biopsied (a photomicrograph of a specimen is shown below) and excised. After her tumor was removed, the woman's symptoms disappeared. The most likely diagnosis is

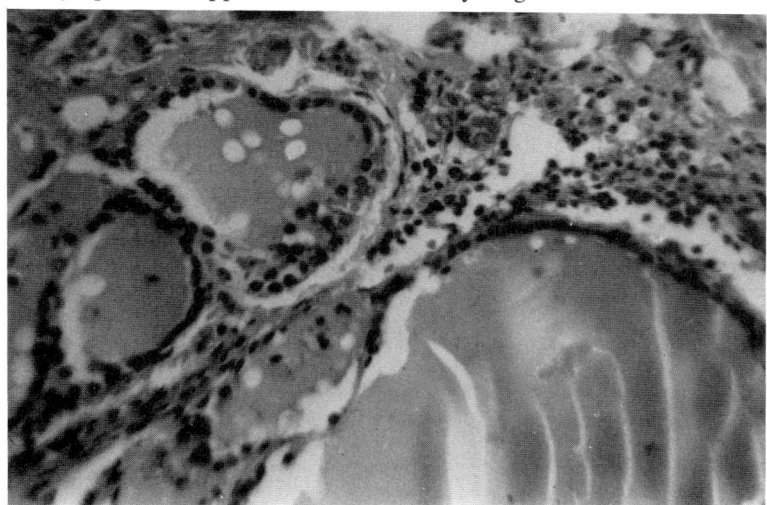

(A) carcinoid tumor
(B) dysgerminoma
(C) embryonal teratoma
(D) endometriosis
(E) struma ovarii

447. A woman is found to have a unilateral, invasive vulvar carcinoma that is 2 cm in diameter but that is not associated with evidence of lymph-node spread. Initial management of this woman most likely would consist of

(A) chemotherapy
(B) radiation therapy
(C) simple vulvectomy
(D) radical vulvectomy
(E) radical vulvectomy and bilateral inguinal lymphadenectomy

448. Most deaths from cervical carcinoma can be attributed to

(A) local extension
(B) metastasis to the central nervous system
(C) metastasis to the liver and lungs
(D) iatrogenic causes
(E) none of the above

449. A 55-year-old woman has a 3-cm raised irregular white lesion at the mucocutaneous junction of the vulva. A sample of the biopsied lesion is shown below. The most likely diagnosis is

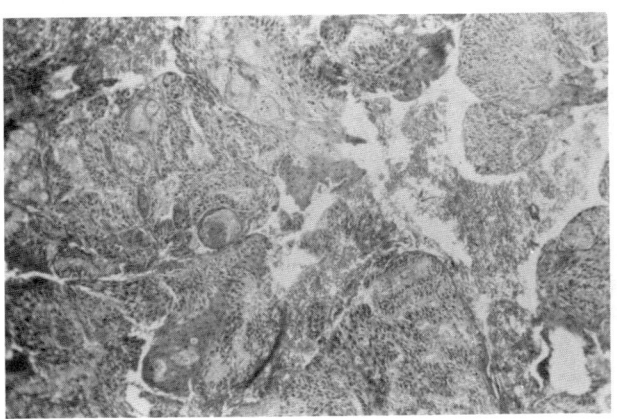

(A) tuberculosis
(B) Bowen's disease
(C) Paget's disease
(D) invasive squamous cell carcinoma
(E) fibrosarcoma

450. Which of the following statements about the International Federation of Gynecology and Obstetrics (FIGO) staging of ovarian carcinoma is true?

(A) Stages I through VI have been defined
(B) Stage II carcinoma is limited to the ovaries
(C) The presence of ascites is significant in differentiating between substages of stage III
(D) Ovarian involvement and spread outside the peritoneal cavity characterize stage IV
(E) The FIGO grouping is based on clinical examination only

451. A 54-year-old woman undergoes a laparotomy because of a pelvic mass, which proves to be a unilateral ovarian neoplasm accompanied by a large omental metastasis. The most appropriate intraoperative course of action would be

(A) omental biopsy
(B) ovarian biopsy
(C) excision of the omental metastasis and unilateral oophorectomy
(D) omentectomy and bilateral salpingo-oophorectomy
(E) omentectomy, total abdominal hysterectomy, and bilateral salpingo-oophorectomy

452. A 45-year-old woman has undergone a total abdominal hysterectomy and bilateral salpingo-oophorectomy for stage II serous carcinoma of the ovary. The most effective postoperative radiotherapeutic treatment of this woman would be

(A) pelvic irradiation
(B) vaginal radium insertion and pelvic irradiation
(C) whole-abdomen irradiation
(D) whole-abdomen and pelvic irradiation
(E) intraperitoneal radioisotope therapy

453. The major mode of spread of ovarian neoplasms is by way of

(A) ovarian veins
(B) ovarian vein lymphatics
(C) pelvic lymphatics
(D) local extension
(E) peritoneal seeding

454. All of the following statements regarding ovarian cancer are true EXCEPT that

(A) it is the most common gynecological cancer
(B) it has the highest mortality rate among the common gynecological cancers
(C) it tends to be asymptomatic until it has reached an advanced stage
(D) its development may be influenced by environmental, cultural, or socioeconomic factors
(E) Papanicolaou (Pap) smears are ineffective for routine diagnostic screening

455. Women who have ovarian carcinoma most commonly present with which of the following symptoms?

(A) Vaginal bleeding and anorexia
(B) Weight loss and dyspareunia
(C) Nausea and vaginal discharge
(D) Constipation and frequent urination
(E) Abdominal distension and pain

456. Mixed mesodermal tumors of the uterus can be described by which of the following statements?

(A) They are more common than previously assumed and comprise about 17 to 18 percent of uterine malignancies
(B) Microscopic examination may reveal the presence of bone, cartilage, muscle, or other elements
(C) Their development has been associated with maternal intake of estrogen during pregnancy
(D) Five-year survival rate is quite good (approximately 80 percent)
(E) They are not known to occur before the menopausal years

457. The class of chemotherapeutic agents that is most effective in the management of women who have recurrent endometrial carcinoma is

(A) antimetabolites
(B) hormones
(C) alkylating agents
(D) Vinca alkaloids
(E) antibiotics

458. The most common sarcoma of the uterus is

(A) endometrial stromal sarcoma
(B) carcinosarcoma
(C) leiomyosarcoma
(D) mixed mesodermal sarcoma
(E) rhabdomyosarcoma

459. Adenoacanthoma of the uterus is considered to represent

(A) a combination malignancy from two separate sources
(B) an adenocarcinoma with squamous metaplasia
(C) an extension of extrauterine adenoacanthoma
(D) a neoplastic transformation of "indifferent" cells beneath normal uterine epithelium
(E) none of the above

460. Young women whose mothers took diethylstilbestrol (DES) during pregnancy are most likely to develop which of the following vaginal carcinomas?

(A) Papillary adenocarcinoma
(B) Squamous carcinoma
(C) Carcinoma of the infantile vagina
(D) Adenosquamous carcinoma
(E) Clear cell adenocarcinoma

461. A 71-year-old woman has postmenopausal bleeding. Fractional dilatation and curettage reveals adenocarcinoma confined to the endometrium. The most important prognostic factor for this woman would be

(A) her age
(B) the tumor grade
(C) the size of her uterus
(D) the depth of myometrial invasion
(E) none of the above

462. Fractional dilatation and curettage reveals endometrial carcinoma involving the cervix. This finding is

(A) of no prognostic significance
(B) of some prognostic significance but does not require change in management
(C) significant only if the cervical tumor is clinically obvious
(D) significant even if the disease is present only microscopically
(E) a contraindication for hysterectomy

463. The primary mode of treatment for endometrial carcinoma confined to the uterine corpus is

(A) external beam radiation
(B) intracavitary radium
(C) hysterectomy
(D) chemotherapy
(E) progestin therapy

464. Women who have endometrial carcinoma most frequently present with which of the following symptoms?

(A) Bloating
(B) Weight loss
(C) Postmenopausal bleeding
(D) Vaginal discharge
(E) Hemoptysis

465. Which of the following statements about carcinoma of the vagina is true?

(A) It most commonly occurs in the lateral walls of the lower one-third of the vagina
(B) Its incidence is highest in women in their sixties and seventies
(C) It is rarely epidermoid
(D) Most affected women have adenocarcinoma
(E) Primary malignancies are more common than secondary malignancies

**DIRECTIONS**: Each question below contains four suggested answers of which **one** or **more** is correct. Choose the answer:

| A | if | 1, 2, and 3 | are correct |
| B | if | 1 and 3 | are correct |
| C | if | 2 and 4 | are correct |
| D | if | 4 | is correct |
| E | if | 1, 2, 3, and 4 | are correct |

466. Meigs' syndrome can be described by which of the following statements?

(1) Hydrothorax and ascites are the primary features
(2) It rarely is seen in combination with ovarian fibromas
(3) It can occur with Brenner tumor, thecoma, and granulosa cell tumor
(4) It characteristically is associated with large subserous myomas

467. Epithelial ovarian tumors of low potential malignancy (borderline malignancies) can be described by which of the following statements?

(1) They represent nearly half of all epithelial ovarian tumors
(2) They occasionally are associated with late recurrences and death
(3) They seldom, if ever, metastasize within the peritoneal cavity
(4) They are not associated with destructive infiltration of the ovarian stroma

468. Epithelial neoplasms of the ovary can be of which of the following histological types?

(1) Serous
(2) Mucinous
(3) Endometrioid
(4) Mesonephroid

469. True statements about myomata uteri include which of the following?

(1) They arise mainly from fibrous tissue
(2) Pedunculation can be seen with submucous or subserous tumors
(3) They rarely cause bleeding
(4) Their excision is the most common indication for hysterectomy

470. Hilus cell tumors of the ovary often are associated with

(1) increased excretion of 17-ketosteroids
(2) elevated levels of plasma testosterone
(3) elevated levels of 17-hydroxycorticoids
(4) hirsutism

471. Dermoid cysts of the ovary can be characterized by which of the following statements?

(1) They often contain bone and teeth, which may be seen on abdominal x-ray
(2) They may be associated with severe chemical peritonitis if ruptured
(3) They are often pedunculated
(4) They are on rare occasions associated with hemolytic anemia

472. True statements regarding myomas of the uterus include which of the following?

(1) They are the most common benign tumors of the uterus
(2) Sarcomatous change is frequent in women over 50 years of age who have myomas
(3) Carneous or red degeneration of myomas occurs frequently during pregnancy
(4) Myomas tend to grow more rapidly after the menopause

473. Carcinoma of the fallopian tube can be described by which of the following statements?

(1) It is an uncommon lesion, accounting for approximately 0.2 to 0.5 percent of primary genital-tract malignancies
(2) Bilateral involvement occurs in approximately 50 percent of affected patients
(3) Its microscopic appearance can be papillary or papillary-alveolar
(4) It is considered only mildly malignant and is associated with a good 5-year survival rate

474. True statements about ovarian neoplasms in children include which of the following?

(1) They are most often of germ cell origin
(2) They are an infrequent cause of precocious puberty
(3) Coelomic epithelial tumors are usually benign
(4) Tumors of germ cell origin are frequently malignant

475. Which of the following statements can characterize epidermoid carcinoma of the vulva?

(1) It is associated with an increased incidence of epidermoid carcinoma of the endocervix
(2) It is seen less frequently than adenocarcinoma
(3) It tends to develop in women who are older than those affected by adenocarcinoma
(4) It tends to be more advanced when diagnosed than adenocarcinoma

476. The disease process illustrated in the slide below can affect which of the following?

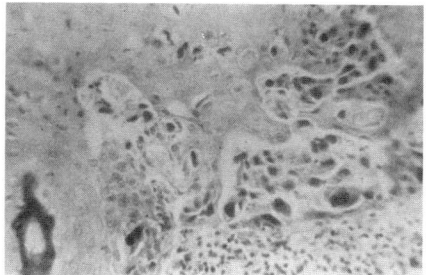

(1) Breast
(2) Cervix
(3) Vulva
(4) Ovary

## SUMMARY OF DIRECTIONS

| A | B | C | D | E |
|---|---|---|---|---|
| 1, 2, 3 only | 1, 3 only | 2, 4 only | 4 only | All are correct |

477. Cervical carcinoma is considered invasive when there is

(1) a breakthrough of the basement membrane
(2) penetration of the stroma
(3) involvement of the lymphatics
(4) involvement of the endocervical glands

478. Vaginal carcinoma in women whose mothers received DES during pregnancy can be characterized by which of the following statements?

(1) It is most commonly located in the middle and outer portions of the vagina
(2) It classically occurs in women in their teens and early twenties
(3) Electron microscopy has shown that it is müllerian in origin
(4) It occurs in less than 0.1 percent of women exposed in utero to DES

479. True statements concerning carcinoma of the vagina include which of the following?

(1) Squamous carcinoma is the most common type
(2) Carcinoma in situ is often multifocal
(3) Metastasis may occur by way of cervical or vulvar lymphatics
(4) Young women are most often affected

480. A woman enters a hospital for an exploratory laparotomy, which reveals the presence of epithelial ovarian cancer. As a result, chemotherapy is begun. Factors that may be of prognostic importance in determining whether this woman will have evidence of disease on a "second look" laparotomy include the

(1) number of courses of chemotherapy
(2) amount of clinically palpable tumor
(3) histological grade of tumor
(4) histological type of epithelial tumor

481. Important prognostic factors concerning ovarian epithelial carcinoma include

(1) extent of the tumor
(2) volume of the tumor
(3) histological differentiation of the tumor
(4) presence of ascites

482. True statements about mucinous carcinoma of the ovary include which of the following?

(1) It usually is diagnosed at a less advanced stage than serous carcinoma
(2) It tends to be unilateral
(3) It tends to be well differentiated
(4) Affected women have a 50-percent chance of surviving 5 years

483. Serous carcinoma of the ovary can be characterized by which of the following statements?

(1) It is the most common epithelial carcinoma of the ovary
(2) It often contains psammoma bodies
(3) It is bilateral in approximately one-third of affected women
(4) It frequently is associated with pelvic endometriosis

484. The spread of adenocarcinoma of the body of the uterus can be described by which of the following statements?

(1) Distant organs, such as the liver, are frequently involved
(2) Dissemination is chiefly by way of the lymphatics
(3) The tumor resembles cervical carcinoma in its frequency of dissemination
(4) Direct extension is an important route of dissemination

485. For the management of women who have endometrial carcinoma, intracavitary radium has been employed routinely

(1) as a treatment for women who have ovarian metastases
(2) as a treatment for women who have vaginal apical recurrences
(3) as a treatment for women who have metastases of the pelvic sidewall
(4) as primary therapy for inoperable patients

486. Sarcoma botryoides can be characterized by which of the following statements?

(1) It tends to be multicentric
(2) Its initial manifestation usually is lower abdominal pain
(3) It occurs most frequently in young girls
(4) Cartilaginous and osseous elements are common

487. Adenocarcinoma of the endometrium can be described by which of the following statements?

(1) It is primarily a disease of postmenopausal women
(2) The average age of affected women is 10 years more than the average age of women who have cervical carcinoma
(3) It has a more favorable prognosis than cervical cancer, with the 5-year survival rate approaching 75 percent
(4) It is increasing in frequency relative to carcinoma of the cervix

488. Evidence in evaluating cell types found in carcinoma of the endometrium suggests that

(1) poorly differentiated adenocarcinomas have a poor prognosis
(2) adenoacanthomas have a poor prognosis
(3) adenosquamous carcinomas have a poor prognosis
(4) adenosquamous tumors occur more often in young women

## SUMMARY OF DIRECTIONS

| A | B | C | D | E |
|---|---|---|---|---|
| 1, 2, 3 only | 1, 3 only | 2, 4 only | 4 only | All are correct |

489. True statements about clear cell adenocarcinoma of the cervix and vagina include which of the following?

(1) It has been related to prenatal DES exposure
(2) It shows a hobnail pattern on microscopic examination
(3) It usually appears as an exophytic lesion
(4) Affected women are best treated with radiotherapy

490. Women who have which of the following characteristics are at high risk for endometrial carcinoma?

(1) Hypertension
(2) Diabetes
(3) Obesity
(4) Familial history of endometrial carcinoma

491. Endometrial adenocarcinoma has been associated with

(1) adenomatous hyperplasia
(2) late menopause
(3) estrogen therapy
(4) multiparity

# Benign and Malignant Neoplasms

**DIRECTIONS:** The groups of questions below consist of lettered choices followed by several numbered items. For each numbered item select the **one** lettered choice with which it is **most** closely associated. Each lettered choice may be used once, more than once, or not at all.

### Questions 492-495

Match the ovarian tumors listed below with the micrograph that correctly exemplifies it.

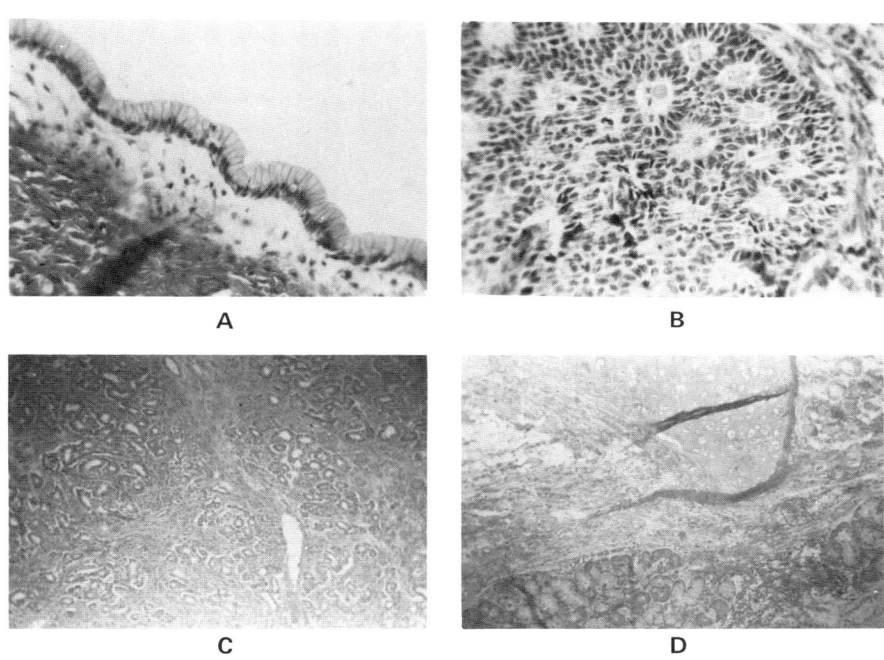

- (A) Slide **A**
- (B) Slide **B**
- (C) Slide **C**
- (D) Slide **D**
- (E) None of the above

492. Granulosa cell tumor

493. Arrhenoblastoma

494. Benign cystic teratoma

495. Mucinous cystadenoma

## Questions 496-500

For each description that follows, select the ovarian tumor with which it is most likely to be associated.

(A) Granulosa tumor
(B) Sertoli-Leydig cell tumor
(C) Immature teratoma
(D) Gonadoblastoma
(E) Krukenberg's tumor

496. Frequently associated with virilization

497. Frequently associated with endometrial carcinoma

498. Tends to recur more than 5 years following the original diagnosis

499. Calcifications present on pelvic radiographs

500. Correlation between malignant potential and the amount of embryogenic tissue

# Benign and Malignant Neoplasms
# Answers

**436. The answer is E.** *(Kistner, ed 3. pp 231-232. Romney, ed 2. p 1085.)* A rapid growth in fibroids (leiomyomas), persistent bleeding, or a fibroid of 12-weeks gestational size or more is considered a valid indication for hysterectomy. Fibroids have a low malignant potential, rarely cause significant pressure when small, and may not cause bleeding problems even when left untreated. They are the most common benign tumors in women and are five times more frequent in blacks than whites.

**437. The answer is B.** *(Kistner, ed 3. p 230.)* If a woman in the childbearing years has an enlarged uterus, a pregnancy test should be performed. Ultrasonography is a more expensive alternative; and an ultrasonogram may be difficult to interpret if both fibroids and an intrauterine pregnancy are present.

**438. The answer is C.** *(Novak, ed 8. pp 120-123.)* Carcinoma in situ (preinvasive cancer) of the cervix involves the entire squamous epithelium, which is displaced by cells that are similar to those of invasive carcinoma. Stratification is completely lost, but no evidence of stromal or lymphatic invasion has been noted. Although carcinoma in situ is generally considered to precede development of frank invasive cancer, the lesion has been reported to regress and disappear on occasion.

**439. The answer is E.** *(Novak, ed 8. pp 441-449.)* Brenner tumors of the ovary, which generally are benign, slow-growing, and asymptomatic, account for 1 to 2 percent of all ovarian neoplasms. Size varies widely; although many are microscopic, some may grow to be quite large (one tumor weighing more than 8.5 kg (19 lb) has been reported). "Walthard rests," which are nests of epithelial cells surrounded by mesenchymal tissue, are diagnostic of Brenner tumor. Nuclei of the epithelial cells are grooved longitudinally and, as a result, are referred to as "coffee-bean" nuclei.

**440. The answer is C.** *(DiSaia, pp 142-144.)* Benign cystic teratomas (dermoid cysts) of the ovary usually appear as anterior cul-de-sac masses that are mobile and unilateral. Serous carcinoma of the ovary, when diagnosed, usually is in an advanced stage and is a fixed, solid mass. Urachal cysts are midline structures and very infrequently diagnosed. Intraligamentous fibroids usually occur in older women, and diverticular abscesses are fixed masses associated with gastrointestinal symptoms.

**441. The answer is A.** *(DiSaia, pp 147-148.)* Ovarian neoplasms arise more commonly from coelomic epithelium than from any other source. Many tumors of this group include epithelium that histologically resembles endocervical, endometrial, or fallopian-tube epithelium (giving rise respectively to mucinous, endometrioid, and serous carcinomas). Other, less common ovarian tumors of coelomic epithelial origin include mesonephroid carcinoma, Brenner tumors, mixed mesodermal tumors, and carcinosarcomas. Epithelial tumors frequently contain mixed cell types; categorization of these tumors is according to the cell type that predominates.

**442. The answer is A.** *(Green, ed 3. pp 126-127.)* Different types of ovarian cancer predominate at different stages of a woman's life. For example, adenocarcinomas, which occur primarily in postmenopausal women, are very rare in infants and children. Benign solid teratomas and especially dermoid cysts, on the other hand, make up about half of the ovarian neoplasms affecting young girls. Giant follicle cysts and theca-lutein cysts also occur rather frequently and presumably are due to maternal gonadotropin stimulation. Granulosa cell tumors, which develop before puberty in about 5 percent of cases, can be a cause of precocious puberty.

**443. The answer is C.** *(Blaustein, p 27. Novak, ed 9. pp 184-186.)* Although rare, adenocarcinoma of Bartholin's gland has to be ruled out in women over 40 years of age who present with Bartholin's cyst. The appropriate treatment in these cases is surgical excision of the Bartholin's gland for a close pathological examination. In cases of abscess formation, both marsupialization of the sac and incision with drainage with appropriate antibiotics are accepted modes of therapy. In the case of the asymptomatic Bartholin's cyst, no treatment is necessary.

**444. The answer is D.** *(Novak, ed 8. p 131.)* The International Federation of Gynecology and Obstetrics (FIGO) classification is the most widely accepted staging for cervical carcinoma. Stage 0 is preinvasive and represents carcinoma in situ. Stage I disease is confined to the cervix; in stage Ia, diagnosis of the malignancy cannot be revealed by clinical examination (stage Ib encompasses all other cases). Although stage II carcinoma extends beyond the cervix, it does not involve the pelvic wall or the lower one-third of the vagina. Obvious parametrial involvement may be absent (stage IIa) or present (stage IIb). Stage III carcinoma extends to the pelvic wall and the lower one-third of the vagina. Stage IV disease extends beyond the true pelvis.

**445. The answer is A.** *(Hilgers, Gynecol Oncol 2:460-475, 1974.)* Gestational trophoblastic disease is the neoplasm most sensitive to appropriate chemotherapeutic agents, such as methotrexate and actinomycin D. Treatment of women who have nonmetastatic gestational trophoblastic disease is almost 100 percent successful and allows reproductive function to be preserved. Cure rates for metastatic disease approach 90 percent.

**446. The answer is E.** *(Novak, ed 8. pp 490-494.)* The tissue specimen that accompanies the question represents struma ovarii, which is composed of aberrant thyroid tissue that is frequently active and which is associated with mature cystic teratomas. The woman described manifests symptoms of thyrotoxicosis, such as diarrhea, rapid pulse, and weight loss; though not reported, her serum thyroxine levels would be elevated. The pathological picture is characterized by thyroid tissue with large acini filled with colloid.

**447. The answer is E.** *(DiSaia, pp 224-226.)* Women who have invasive vulvar carcinoma usually are treated surgically. If the lesions are unilateral, are not associated with fixed or ulcerated inguinal lymph nodes, and do not involve the urethra, vagina, anus, or rectum, then treatment usually consists of radical vulvectomy and bilateral inguinal lymphadenectomy. If inguinal lymph nodes show evidence of metastatic disease, bilateral pelvic lymphadenectomy is usually performed. Radiation therapy, though not a routine part of the management of women who have early vulvar carcinoma, is employed (as an alternative to pelvic exenteration with radical vulvectomy) in the treatment of women who have local advanced carcinoma.

**448. The answer is A.** *(Novak, ed 8. p 130.)* Most deaths from cervical cancer result from the effects of local extension. These effects include urinary insufficiency, intestinal obstruction, and debility and malnutrition. Approximately two-fifths of all women who die of cervical cancer have evidence of extrapelvic metastasis; spread of the tumor, presumably via the bloodstream, occasionally involves distant organs, including the liver, spine, and brain.

**449. The answer is D.** *(Novak, ed 8. pp 43-48.)* The woman described in the question has invasive squamous cell carcinoma of the vulva, with penetration below the basement membrane. The squamous epithelial cells have an irregular shape and an abnormal nuclear-cytoplasmic ratio and show an increased number of mitotic figures. Tuberculosis of the vulva is characterized by multinucleated giant cells; Bowen's disease tissue does not show invasion below the basement membrane; and Paget's disease of the vulva, which is rare, is characterized by Paget cells, large cells that have abundant granular cytoplasm and basophilic nuclei.

**450. The answer is D.** *(DiSaia, p 11.)* The FIGO staging of primary ovarian carcinoma is in four categories: stage I (with substages a to c), in which growth is limited to one or both ovaries and in which ascites can be present (stage Ic); stage II (with substages a, b, and c), in which carcinoma shows pelvic extension; stage III, in which intraperitoneal metastasis is widespread; and stage IV, in which the cancer has metastasized outside the peritoneal cavity. Disease that is thought to be, but not proven to be, ovarian carcinoma is defined as a special category. The FIGO staging is based on both clinical examination and surgical exploration.

**451. The answer is E.** *(DiSaia, p 164.)* The survivability of women who have ovarian carcinoma varies inversely with the amount of residual tumor left after the initial surgery. At the time of laparotomy, a maximum effort should be made to determine the sites of tumor spread and excise all resectable tumor. Although the uterus and ovary may appear grossly normal, there is a relatively high incidence of occult metastases to these organs; for this reason, they should be removed during the initial surgery.

**452. The answer is D.** *(Rutledge, pp 188-189.)* Postoperative whole-abdomen irradiation combined with additional radiation to the pelvis has produced the highest 5-year survival rates of any treatment used for patients who have stage II epithelial ovarian tumors. Because ovarian tumor cells tend to exfoliate and spread throughout the abdominal cavity, irradiation of the pelvis alone is insufficient treatment. The liver and kidneys must be shielded during at least part of the external beam therapy, and bowel injury may be a late sequela.

**453. The answer is E.** *(Rutledge, pp 164-166.)* Peritoneal seeding is the major mode of spread of ovarian neoplasms. Ovarian malignancies also may extend locally to adjoining structures, such as the uterus, fallopian tubes, pelvic peritoneum, bladder peritoneum, and serosa of the sigmoid colon. Although dissemination by lymphatic and hematogenous routes does occur, it is of lesser importance than peritoneal seeding in producing symptoms and eventually causing death.

**454. The answer is A.** *(Rutledge, pp 159-160, 162.)* Ovarian carcinoma, though the third most common malignancy of gynecological origin (after endometrial and cervical carcinoma), is associated with the highest mortality rate among the common gynecological malignancies. The inability of routine screening tests to diagnose this malignancy in an early stage, in contrast to the efficacy of the Papanicolaou (Pap) smear in detecting cervical cancer, is chiefly responsible for the high mortality rate. Most patients have advanced disease by the time their symptoms appear. Environmental, cultural, socioeconomic, and dietary factors all may play a role in the development of ovarian cancer.

**455. The answer is E.** *(DiSaia, p 140.)* Approximately 70 percent of women who have ovarian cancer present with abdominal distension, and 50 percent present with abdominal pain. Gastrointestinal symptoms, which occur in about 20 percent of affected women, often are secondary to the development of ascites. Urinary-tract symptoms, due to the pressure exerted by a rapidly growing mass, and abnormal vaginal bleeding are the initial symptoms of ovarian cancer in 15 percent of affected women.

**456. The answer is B.** *(Novak, ed 8. pp 300-304.)* Mixed mesodermal tumors (mesenchymomas) of the uterus are similar to endometrial sarcoma. They are made up of a composite of mesodermal elements such as bone, cartilage, and muscle. The combined incidence of these two types of malignancy is no higher than 0.5 percent of all gynecological malignancies. Although mixed mesodermal tumors occur most frequently in postmenopausal women, one variant, sarcoma botryoides, can develop in young children. Prognosis is poor, with a 5-year survival rate of 26 to 28 percent being the highest reported. Maternal ingestion of estrogen during pregnancy has not, as yet, been associated with the development of mixed mesodermal tumors.

**457. The answer is B.** *(Rutledge, pp 124-128.)* Progestins have been employed successfully in the treatment of women who have recurrent endometrial carcinoma. In many series, response rates of 30 to 40 percent have been noted. The most frequently employed agents have been hydroxyprogesterone caproate (Delalutin) and medroxyprogesterone acetate (Provera). Single-agent chemotherapy with nonhormonal agents has produced disappointing responses in patients affected by advanced or recurrent endometrial carcinoma.

**458. The answer is C.** *(Rutledge, p 132.)* Leiomyosarcomas are the most common sarcomas of the uterus. They are discovered most frequently during a histological examination of a leiomyomatous uterus and are often clinically and grossly indistinguishable from benign leiomyoma. A rapid enlargement of a leiomyomatous uterus may be the only indication of the presence of a sarcoma.

**459. The answer is B.** *(Novak, ed 8. pp 214-215.)* The belief that adenoacanthoma of the uterus is a combination of malignant tumors generally has been discarded. Current investigators feel that this tumor represents an adenocarcinoma with squamous metaplastic changes. When compared stage to stage, adenoacanthoma and adenocarcinoma have similar prognoses.

**460. The answer is E.** *(Rutledge, pp 262-264.)* Young women whose mothers ingested diethylstilbestrol (DES) during pregnancy are more apt to develop clear cell adenocarcinoma than other types of vaginal carcinoma. Although squamous carcinomas are the most common tumors of the vagina, they usually occur in women over 40 years of age. Two rare vaginal carcinomas are papillary adenocarcinoma, which primarily affects older women, and carcinoma of the infantile vagina, which histologically resembles an endodermal sinus tumor of the ovary. Adenosquamous carcinomas usually are found in the uterus and less frequently in the cervix.

**461. The answer is B.** *(DiSaia, pp 114-116.)* The most important prognostic factor for stage I endometrial carcinoma (carcinoma confined to the corpus uteri) is the grade, or degree of differentiation, of the tumor. Grade 1 tumors are well differentiated and are associated with a 5-year survival rate of greater than 80 percent; grade 3 tumors are poorly differentiated and are associated with a 5-year survival rate of less than 45 percent. The depth of myometrial invasion and the involvement of pelvic lymph nodes correlate inversely with the degree of differentiation. Older women tend to have less well-differentiated tumors and therefore a poorer chance of survival.

**462. The answer is D.** *(Rutledge, pp 99-100, 110.)* Endometrial carcinoma involving the cervix is significant even if present only as microscopic disease. The lymphatic drainage of the uterine corpus is primarily by way of the lymphatics that follow the ovarian vessels. Because involvement of the cervix allows the cancer to metastasize via the parametrial lymphatics, 5-year survival rate is reduced (regardless of the volume of tumor present) and intense radiotherapeutic treatment is required. Hysterectomy need not be excluded from the management program.

**463. The answer is C.** *(Rutledge, pp 106-107.)* Hysterectomy is the primary mode of treatment for women who have endometrial carcinoma confined to the uterine corpus. External beam and intracavitary radiation have been employed to help reduce central and pelvic recurrences of the cancer. Progestin therapy is used routinely as primary treatment of women who have advanced disease or recurrent carcinoma, and chemotherapy is used for patients whose tumors have failed to respond to other forms of therapy.

**464. The answer is C.** *(Brady, Gynecol Oncol 2:314-323, 1974.)* Postmenopausal bleeding is the most common presenting symptom of women who have endometrial carcinoma. Because this warning signal is present even in the earliest stage of the disease, early diagnosis and treatment are possible. In fact, approximately 70 percent of affected women have stage I disease when they first seek treatment.

**465. The answer is B.** *(Novak, ed 8. pp 70-74.)* Carcinoma of the vagina, which occurs most frequently in women in their sixties and seventies, is most commonly epidermoid in origin and only rarely takes the form of adenocarcinoma. In addition, secondary carcinoma occurs much more frequently than primary carcinoma. The upper half of the anterior and posterior vaginal walls is most apt to be the site of vaginal carcinoma.

**466. The answer is B (1, 3).** *(Novak, ed 8. pp 451-454.)* Hydrothorax and ascites are the characteristic features of Meigs' syndrome. It is believed that fluid accumulates in the thorax by permeating through diaphragmatic lymphatics. First described in association with ovarian fibromas, Meigs' syndrome also can be seen in combination with Brenner tumors, thecomas, granulosa cell tumors, and other solid ovarian tumors; large subserous myomas, however, are not associated with development of this syndrome.

**467. The answer is C (2, 4).** *(DiSaia, pp 153-157.)* Epithelial ovarian tumors of low potential malignancy represent 15 percent of all epithelial ovarian tumors. Although they do not infiltrate destructively into the ovarian stroma, these borderline malignancies have been associated with late recurrences and death and may metastasize throughout the peritoneal cavity. Histologically, these tumors demonstrate proliferative activity, abnormal mitoses, and nuclear abnormalities. Ten-year survival rates of women who have stage I tumors of low potential malignancy have been reported to be 95 percent.

**468. The answer is E (all).** *(Novak, ed 8. pp 396-435.)* Epithelial neoplasms, which comprise 75 to 80 percent of all primary ovarian cancers, may be of the following histological types: serous, mucinous, endometrioid, and mesonephroid. These types may be thought of as forms of differentiated mesotheliomas. Serous lesions are the most common variety of ovarian cystomas. Mucinous tumors may become large enough to fill the abdomen. The prognosis is good for women who have endometrioid lesions, which metastasize only infrequently, and are not considered to be very malignant. Pure mesonephroid tumors are rare.

**469. The answer is C (2, 4).** *(Mattingly, ed 5. pp 187-194.)* Myomata uteri (uterine fibroids) arise from fibromuscular tissue, with more smooth muscle than fibrous tissue present. All myomata uteri arise in the myometrium; and although they initially occur interstitially, they can grow internally (submucous lesions) or externally (subserous) and become pedunculated. Myomata uteri, which frequently cause bleeding, are the most common uterine tumors; their excision, not surprisingly, is the most common indication for hysterectomy.

**470. The answer is C (2, 4).** *(Green, ed 3. p 190.)* Hilus cell (pure Leydig cell) tumors are small, unilateral tumors of the ovary. They cause hirsutism and virilization by production of testosterone; levels of 17-hydroxycorticoids and excretion of 17-ketosteroids are not usually increased. Hyperplasia and luteinization of the ovarian stroma often occur and lead to endometrial hyperplasia (in contrast to endometrial atrophy that often accompanies arrhenoblastomas).

**471. The answer is E (all).** *(Green, ed 3. pp 476-477.)* Dermoid cysts are characteristically pedunculated, which predisposes them to undergo tension, one of the more common complications associated with this tumor. It has been estimated that teeth, which are visible on abdominal x-ray, are present in approximately 50 percent of cases. When the dermoid cyst is ruptured, the contents are extremely irritating to the peritoneum and incite an intense granulomatous inflammatory reaction. Hemolytic anemia has been reported as one of the complications; it resolves completely on surgical removal of the dermoid cyst.

**472. The answer is B (1, 3).** *(Green, ed 3. pp 381-382, 385-387.)* Myomas are indeed the most common benign gynecological tumor in women. It has been estimated that approximately 20 to 30 percent of all women will develop this tumor during their lifetime, with many of them remaining completely asymptomatic. The incidence has been shown to be higher in black women for-yet-unknown reasons. Sarcomatous changes are infrequent, being in the range of approximately 0.5 percent. Red or carneous degeneration of myomas occurs especially during pregnancy, when the high levels of estrogen stimulate rapid growth of the tumor, resulting in impairment of the vascular supply, especially to the center of the tumor. Clinically, it is important to distinguish between this entity and other possible causes of abdominal pain in pregnancy since conservative supportive therapy usually suffices in the case of red degeneration of myomas. Following the menopause, the myomas usually decrease in size because of decreased estrogen levels.

**473. The answer is B (1, 3).** *(Novak, ed 8. pp 335-341.)* Because affected women have a low 5-year survival rate, primary tubal carcinoma is thought to be highly malignant; this relationship, however, may be due more to delayed discovery of the tumor than to its malignant potential. Primary tubal carcinoma accounts for only 0.2 to 0.5 percent of primary malignancies of the genital tract. Microscopically, these tumors present a papillary or papillary-alveolar pattern. Bilateral involvement occurs in about one-fourth of affected women.

**474. The answer is E (all).** *(DiSaia, p 189.)* Most ovarian neoplasms in children are of germ cell origin, and about half of these tumors are malignant. Functioning ovarian tumors have been reported to produce precocious puberty in about 2 percent of affected patients. Epithelial tumors of the ovary, which are quite rare in prepubertal girls, are benign in approximately 90 percent of all cases.

**475. The answer is B (1, 3).** *(DiSaia, pp 227-228.)* Epidermoid carcinoma, the most common variety of vulvar cancer, usually is diagnosed at a less advanced stage than adenocarcinoma, which is a rare tumor that most often arises from Bartholin's glands. Epidermoid carcinoma tends to affect women who, on the average, are older than those affected by adenocarcinoma. Women who have epidermoid carcinoma of the vulva have been noted to have an increased incidence of epidermoid carcinoma of the cervix.

**476. The answer is B (1, 3).** *(Novak, ed 8. pp 40-42. Romney, ed 2. pp 1011, 1197-1198.)* The lesion illustrated in the question is characteristic of Paget's disease. Paget cells are large and vacuolated, with a distinct, basophilic nucleus. Paget's disease is a carcinoma of apocrine sweat glands, which are found in the vulva and areola of the breast. The vulvar form presents grossly as a reddish lesion interspersed with white epithelial islands. While the breast lesion often has underlying carcinoma, vulvar Paget's disease is usually in situ. Treatment for women who have vulvar Paget's disease is vulvectomy. Women with lymph node metastases have a very poor prognosis, and treatment in these cases includes radical groin dissection.

**477. The answer is A (1, 2, 3).** *(Novak, ed 8. pp 123-129.)* Carcinoma of the cervix is considered to be invasive when the basement membrane has been pierced, allowing cancer cells into the stroma. Histological evidence of abnormal cell maturation and presence of cancer cells in the lymphatics also indicate invasive disease. Involvement of endocervical glands is not indicative of invasion.

**478. The answer is E (all).** *(Novak, ed 8. pp 73-74.)* A number of young women whose mothers were treated with DES during pregnancy (particularly before the eighteenth week of gestation) have been found to have adenocarcinoma of the vagina. The tumors of these women, who generally are in their late teens or early twenties, usually are located in the middle third or outer third of the vagina. Microscopic examination reveals that the malignancies are clear cell tumors with papillary projections; when viewed by electron microscopy, these tumors show evidence of a müllerian origin.

**479. The answer is A (1, 2, 3).** *(Rutledge, pp 259-260.)* Squamous carcinoma of the vagina, which tends to occur in older women and is most frequently located on the posterior wall of the vagina, is the most common type of vaginal carcinoma. Carcinoma in the lower one-third of the vagina can metastasize by way of vulvar lymphatics; tumors situated in the upper vagina may spread via cervical lymphatics. Carcinoma in situ of the vagina is often multifocal.

**480. The answer is A (1, 2, 3).** *(Rutledge, pp 194-197.)* The histological type of epithelial ovarian cancer does not appear to play a significant role in the progression or regression of disease between initial and "second look" surgery. Factors that are of prognostic significance include the volume of residual tumor left at the initial surgery, the number of courses of chemotherapy, and the presence of palpable tumor. The histological grade of the initial tumor also is prognostically significant, because women who have well-differentiated tumors appear to respond better to chemotherapy than women affected by poorly differentiated tumors.

**481. The answer is E (all).** *(DiSaia, pp 161-164.)* The extent (or stage) and the volume of a tumor are probably the most important prognostic considerations in the management of women who have ovarian epithelial carcinoma. However, on a stage-for-stage basis, women who have well-differentiated tumors have better prognoses than women who have poorly differentiated tumors. The presence of ascites or peritoneal washings that are cytologically positive for malignant cells decreases the 5-year survival of affected women.

**482. The answer is E (all).** *(Rutledge, pp 167-169.)* Mucinous carcinomas of the ovary usually are diagnosed at an earlier stage than serous carcinomas and tend to be histologically well differentiated. This combination of diagnosis at an early stage (when the tumors frequently are unilateral) and well-differentiated histological appearance is probably the reason that women who have mucinous carcinoma have a better 5-year survival rate than women affected by serous carcinoma. Mucinous tumors of the ovary, which are less common than serous lesions, usually are lobulated and may grow to enormous proportions.

**483. The answer is A (1, 2, 3).** *(DiSaia, pp 157-160.)* Serous carcinoma is the most common epithelial tumor of the ovary. Psammoma bodies can be seen in approximately 30 percent of these tumors; and bilateral involvement characterizes about one-third of all serous carcinomas. Although mesonephroid carcinomas tend to be associated with pelvic endometriosis, a similar association has not been demonstrated for serous carcinomas.

**484. The answer is C (2, 4).** *(Novak, ed 8. p 219.)* Although the most common route of dissemination of adenocarcinoma of the body of the uterus is the lymphatics, this tumor spreads much less often than cervical malignancies and only rarely affects distant organs. Nearby surface structures are affected more frequently, and the cervix, bladder, and rectum can become involved in advanced cases. Direct extension, though not as common as lymphatic dissemination, also is important.

**485. The answer is C (2, 4).** *(Brady, Gynecol Oncol 2:314-323, 1974.)* Intracavitary radium has been successfully employed as the primary mode of therapy for women who have surgically inoperable endometrial cancer and have small uteri with a well-differentiated tumor. Vaginal apical recurrences occur in 10 to 15 percent of affected women who were treated by hysterectomy alone; this incidence can be reduced significantly with the use of intravaginal radium. Because the effectiveness of intracavitary radium rapidly decreases as tissue depth increases, it is not a satisfactory treatment for women who have ovarian or pelvic sidewall metastases.

**486. The answer is B (1, 3).** *(DiSaia, pp 212-213. Romney, ed 2. p 379.)* Sarcoma botryoides, a rare and highly malignant tumor, is characterized grossly by a polypoid mass that can expand to occupy the entire vagina and frequently protrudes through the vaginal introitus. The usual presenting symptom is vaginal discharge or bleeding. Sarcoma botryoides, which occurs most frequently in young girls, is usually multicentric in origin. Cartilagenous and osseous elements are not commonly found, although rhabdomyoblastic elements are. Extensive surgery (extenteration), without which death will result, can extend the survival rate to several years.

**487. The answer is E (all).** *(Novak, ed 8. pp 204-205.)* Although the carcinogenesis of endometrial cancer is still in dispute, several facts regarding its incidence are clear. The disease primarily affects women who have passed the menopause; on the average, endometrial cancer appears 10 years later than the onset of cervical carcinoma. The fact that the frequency of this condition has been increasing certainly is due in part to the increased life span of American women. Most studies have revealed a 5-year survival rate of about 75 percent for women who have endometrial cancer.

**488. The answer is B (1, 3).** *(Rutledge, p 101.)* Recent evidence suggests that adenosquamous carcinoma of the endometrium has a poorer prognosis than either adenocarcinoma or adenoacanthoma of the endometrium. It has yet to be resolved whether the poorer prognosis associated with adenosquamous lesions is due to the population of malignant squamous cells or to the poorly differentiated adenomatous elements, which normally carry a poor prognosis. Adenoacanthoma, which is characterized by benign metaplasia of squamous epithelium, has a prognosis similar to that of other adenocarcinomas of the endometrium. Adenosquamous tumors tend to occur more frequently in older women.

**489. The answer is A (1, 2, 3).** *(Green, ed 3. pp 128-131.)* In the late 1960s, a surprisingly large number of cases of a rare type of clear cell adenocarcinoma of the cervix and vagina were discovered in Boston. Careful epidemiological investigation revealed that nearly all the mothers of affected girls had taken DES or a similar drug during pregnancy. These tumors are exophytic lesions that are friable and red. Microscopic examination characteristically reveals the presence of cystic spaces lined with so-called hobnail cells. Because affected women usually are in their adolescence and because the tumors are relatively radioresistant, surgery has been the main component of management.

**490. The answer is E (all).** *(MacMahon, Gynecol Oncol 2:122-129, 1974.)* Endometrial carcinoma tends to occur in obese, diabetic women who undergo late-onset menopause and are nulliparous or have low parity. Other factors that may predispose to endometrial carcinoma include hypertension, cancer at other sites (e.g., ovary and breast), and familial history of this malignancy.

**491. The answer is A (1, 2, 3).** *(Novak, ed 8. pp 220-229.)* Adenocarcinoma of the uterus has been found to be associated with such gynecological factors as late menopause, anovulation, and a poor fertility index. Prolonged estrogen therapy, too, has been implicated in the development of uterine cancer. Adenomatous hyperplasia of the endometrium is not only associated with adenocarcinoma but also widely considered to be a precancerous lesion.

**492-495. The answers are: 492-B, 493-C, 494-D, 495-A.** *(Novak, ed 8. pp 409-416, 485-490, 505-511, 523-530.)* Granulosa cell tumors show considerable microscopic variation. In most instances constituent cells resemble granulosa cells; and Call-Exner bodies, which are small liquefied cysts common in granulosa cells, may be observed in the better-differentiated forms of the tumor.

Arrhenoblastomas are malignant, masculinizing ovarian tumors. Testicular structures may be present (in the accompanying micrograph, testicularlike tubules can be observed). Reinke crystalloids also are often noted.

Benign cystic teratomas are the most common type of ovarian teratoma. The presence of sebaceous glandular elements are common; bone, cartilage, hair follicles, and skin also are frequently encountered.

Mucinous cystadenomas are characterized by the presence of the familiar, columnar, mucin-producing cells lining the cyst cavity. No evidence of malignancy typically is found.

**496-500. The answers are: 496-B, 497-A, 498-A, 499-D, 500-C.** *(DiSaia, pp 176-177, 181-185. Romney, ed 2. p 1167. Rutledge, pp 206-207.)* Sertoli-Leydig cell tumors, which represent less than 1 percent of ovarian tumors, may produce symptoms of virilization. Histologically, they resemble fetal testes; clinically, they must be distinguished from other functioning ovarian neoplasms as well as from tumors of the adrenal glands. Recurrences of Sertoli-Leydig cell tumors, which seem to have a low malignant potential, usually appear within 3 years of the original diagnosis.

Granulosa and theca cell tumors often are associated with excessive estrogen production, which may cause pseudoprecocious puberty, postmenopausal bleeding, or menorrhagia. These tumors are associated with endometrial carcinoma in 15 percent of patients. Because these tumors are quite friable, affected women frequently present with symptoms caused by tumor rupture and intraperitoneal bleeding. Granulosa tumors are low-grade malignancies that tend to recur more than 5 years after the initial diagnosis. Because their malignant potential is impossible to predict histologically, long-term follow-up is mandatory for these patients. Recurrences have been reported as late as 33 years after the original diagnosis.

Gonadoblastomas frequently contain calcifications that can be detected by plain radiography of the pelvis. Women who have gonadoblastomas often have ambiguous genitalia. The tumors are usually small and, in one-third of affected women, bilateral.

The malignant potential of immature teratomas correlates with the degree of immature or embryonic tissue present. The presence of choriocarcinoma can be determined histologically as well as by human chorionic gonadotropin (HCG) assays. The presence of choriocarcinoma in an immature teratoma worsens the prognosis.

Krukenberg's tumors are typically bilateral, solid masses of the ovary that nearly always represent metastases from another organ, usually the stomach. They contain large numbers of signet-ring adenocarcinoma cells within a cellular hyperplastic but non-neoplastic ovarian stroma.

# Bibliography

Adamsons K Jr, Joelsson I: The effects of pharmacologic agents upon the fetus and newborn. *Am J Obstet Gynecol* 96:437-460, 1966.

Aladjem S, Brown AK (eds): *Clinical Perinatology,* 2nd ed. St. Louis, CV Mosby, 1979.

American College of Obstetricians and Gynecologists: Suspect rape. *Am Coll Obstet Gynecol Tech Bull* 14:July, 1972.

American Medical Association Committee on Human Sexuality: *Human Sexuality:* Chicago, American Medical Association, 1972.

Barden TP, Peter JB, Merkatz IR: Ritodrine hydrochloride: a betamimetic agent for use in preterm labor. I. Pharmacology, clinical history, administration, side effects, and safety. *Obstet Gynecol* 56:1-6, 1980.

Beck WS: *Hematology,* 2nd ed. Cambridge, MIT Press, 1977.

Behrman SJ, Kistner RW (eds): *Progress in Infertility,* 2nd ed. Boston, Little, Brown, 1975.

Benirschke K: Twin placenta in perinatal mortality. *NY State J Med* 61:4499-4508, 1961.

Blaustein A (ed): *Pathology of the Female Genital Tract.* New York, Springer-Verlag, 1977.

Brady LW, Lewis GC, Antoniades J, et al: Evolution of radiotherapeutic techniques. *Gynecol Oncol* 2:314-323, 1974.

Burrow GN, Ferris TF (eds): *Medical Complications During Pregnancy.* Philadelphia, WB Saunders, 1975.

Butler NR, Goldstein H, Ross EM: Cigarette smoking in pregnancy: its influence on birth weight and perinatal mortality. *Br Med J* 2:127-130, 1972.

Dickinson RL: *Human Sex Anatomy.* Melbourne, Fla., RE Krieger Publishing, 1949.

Dickinson RL, Pierson HH: The average sex life of American women. *JAMA* 85:1113-1117, 1925.

DiSaia PJ, Morrow CP, Townsend DE: *Synopsis of Gynecologic Oncology.* New York, John Wiley & Sons, 1975.

Ellenberg M: Impotence in diabetics: the neurologic factor. *Ann Intern Med* 75:213-219, 1971.

Gilman AG, et al (eds): *The Pharmacological Basis of Therapeutics,* 6th ed. New York, Macmillan, 1980.

Golbus MS: The antenatal detection of genetic disorders. Current status and future prospects. *Obstet Gynecol* 48:497-506, 1976.

Green R: *Human Sexuality,* 2nd ed. Baltimore, Williams & Wilkins, 1979.

Green TH Jr: *Gynecology: Essentials of Clinical Practice,* 3rd ed. Boston, Little, Brown, 1977.

Herbst AL, Scully RE, Robboy SJ: Vaginal adenosis and other diethylstilbestrol-related abnormalities. *Clin Obstet Gynecol* 18:185-194, 1975.

Hilgers RD, Lewis JL: Gestational trophoblastic neoplasms. *Gynecol Oncol* 2:460-475, 1974.

Hon EH: *An Atlas of Fetal Heart Rate Patterns.* New Haven, Harty Press, 1968.

Ingemarsson I: Effect of terbutaline on premature labor. A double-blind placebo-controlled study. *Am J Obstet Gynecol* 125:520-524, 1976.

Isselbacher KJ, et al (eds): *Harrison's Principles of Internal Medicine,* 9th ed. New York, McGraw-Hill, 1980.

Jeffcoate N: *Principles of Gynecology,* 4th ed. Woburn, Mass., Butterworth, 1975.

Kistner RW: *Gynecology: Principles and Practice,* 3rd ed. Chicago, Year Book Medical, 1978.

Kolodny RC: Sexual dysfunction in diabetic females. *Diabetes* 20:557-559, 1971.

Ledger WJ: Antibiotics in pregnancy: classes of antibiotics prescribed to pregnant women. *Clin Obstet Gynecol* 20:417-418, 1977.

Lief HI: *Medical Aspects of Human Sexuality: Answers to Questions by 502 Authorities.* Baltimore, Williams & Wilkins, 1975.

MacMahon B: High risk factors for endometrial cancer. *Gynecol Oncol* 2:122-129, 1974.

Masters WH, Johnson VE: *Human Sexual Inadequacy.* Boston, Little, Brown, 1970.

Masters WH, Johnson VE: *Human Sexual Response.* Boston, Little, Brown, 1966.

Mattingly RF: *Te Linde's Operative Gynecology,* 5th ed. New York, JB Lippincott, 1977.

McCrann DJ, Schifrin BS: Fetal monitoring in high risk pregnancy. *Clin Perinatol* 1:229-252, 1974.

Mishell DR Jr, Davajan V: *Reproductive Endocrinology, Infertility and Contraception.* Philadelphia, FA Davis, 1979.

Monif GR (ed): *Infectious Diseases in Obstetrics and Gynecology.* Hagerstown, Harper & Row, 1974.

Nahmias AJ: Perinatal risk associated with maternal genetic herpes simplex virus infection. *Am J Obstet Gynecol* 110:825, 1971.

NICHD National Registry for Amniocentesis Study Group: Midtrimester amniocentesis for prenatal diagnosis. *JAMA* 236:1471-1476, 1976.

Novak ER: *Textbook of Gynaecology,* 9th ed. Baltimore, Williams & Wilkins, 1975.

Novak ER, Woodruff JD: *Novak's Gynecologic and Obstetric Pathology: With Clinical and Endocrine Relations,* 8th ed. Philadelphia, WB Saunders, 1979.

Parsons L, Sommers SC: *Gynecology,* 2nd ed. Philadelphia, WB Saunders, 1978.

Peck TM, Arias F: Hematologic changes associated with pregnancy. *Clin Obstet Gynecol* 22:785-789, 1979.

Pritchard JA, MacDonald PC: *Williams Obstetrics,* 16th ed. New York, Appleton-Century-Crofts, 1980.

Queenan JT: *Modern Management of the Rh Problem,* 2nd ed. Hagerstown, Harper & Row, 1977.

Ratnoff OD (ed): *Treatment of Hemorrhagic Disorders.* Hagerstown, Harper & Row, 1968.

Reid DE, et al: *Principles and Management of Human Reproduction.* Philadelphia, WB Saunders, 1972.

Robertson JG: Twin pregnancy: morbidity and fetal mortality. *Obstet Gynecol* 23:330-337, 1964.

Romney SL, et al (eds): *Gynecology and Obstetrics: The Health Care of Women,* 2nd ed. New York, McGraw-Hill, 1981.

Rutledge F, Boronow RC, Wharton JT: *Gynecologic Oncology.* New York, John Wiley & Sons, 1976.

Ryan GM Jr (ed): *Ambulatory Care in Obstetrics and Gynecology.* New York, Grune & Stratton, 1980.

Sciarra JJ (ed): *Gynecology and Obstetrics.* Hagerstown, Harper & Row, 1977.

Scott JR: Report on Rh immune globulin therapy. *Contemp Obstet Gynecol* 8:27, 1976.

Speroff L, Glass RH, Kase NG: *Clinical Gynecologic Endocrinology and Infertility,* 2nd ed. Baltimore, Williams & Wilkins, 1978.

Thompson JS, Thompson MW: *Genetics in Medicine,* 3rd ed. Philadelphia, WB Saunders, 1980.

U.S. Department of Health, Education and Welfare: # (PHS) 79-50066:11-43, 1979.

Villee CA, Villee DB, Zuckerman A: *Respiratory Distress Syndrome: Based on a Conference at Dedham, Mass. May 1973.* New York, Academic Press, 1973.

Williams RH (ed): *Textbook of Endocrinology,* 5th ed. Philadelphia, WB Saunders, 1974.

Willson JR, Carrington ER: *Obstetrics and Gynecology,* 6th ed. St. Louis, CV Mosby, 1979.

Working Party on Amniocentesis: *Br J Obstet Gynaecol* 185:2, 1978.

Wynn RM: *Obstetrics and Gynecology: The Clinical Core,* 2nd ed. Philadelphia, Lea & Febiger, 1979.

Yen SS, Jaffe RB (eds): *Reproductive Endocrinology: Physiology, Pathophysiology and Clinical Management.* Philadelphia, WB Saunders, 1978.

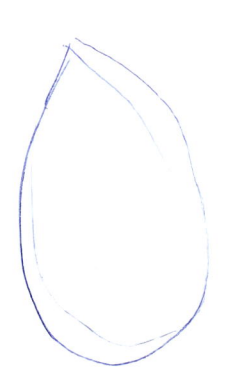